If You Think You Don't Have PTSD,
THINK AGAIN!

The World's First Research-Backed, Drug-Free Remedy for the
Global PTSD Pandemic Stress Syndrome

By Dr. Jamie Turndorf

Praise

"In one Energetic System Upgrade™ with Dr. Jamie an issue that's been nagging at me for 30 years is 80% gone."

— Dr. Sherri J. Tenpenny,
Osteopathic Medical Doctor, Board-Certified
in Three Medical Specialties

"Dr. Jamie Turndorf puts together an excellent resource for those trying to understand how PTSD manifests itself in many people who do not understand its nature and, therefore, do not fi nd the appropriate therapy for their health issues. Her book is an excellent source of information for all those questioning their emotional and physical health issues."

— Bernie Siegel, MD author of *No Endings Only Beginnings and Love Medicine & Miracles*

"I am so thrilled that Dr. Jamie Turndorf decided to write this excellent book about how we can better manage our own mental health recovery from excessive stress and PTSD. It's time to take charge and be proactive. Don't wait for someone to give you a magic pill to fix the ill. Th at is just a fantasy. Everyone needs this information now more than ever to recover from the devas-tating effects of unrelenting environmental stress plaguing our modern world. Find out what kind of nutritional deficiency can deplete the Central Nervous System. Learn what you can do to refill your tank and to rebuild and recover your mojo and energy supply. Make yourself strong from the inside out. Recharge your batteries and enjoy a fulfilling life again. There is no need to put up with chronic anxiety, depression, sleep disorders, mood swings, brain fog, sexual dysfunction, headaches or other body pains. It's not natural. The good news is that nature provides us with knight-in-shining-armour nutrition that can rescue us from that downward slide. It's really not rocket science, just simple nutritional know-how. This book is literally a lifesaver. Follow Dr. Jamie's advice right now. Your life literally depends on it.

— Sandy Sanderson

Today we live in a complicated world where human health and well-being are constantly under attack. While we have advanced technology at our disposal, we still suffer from all kinds of diseases, not realizing that excessive stress and PTSD could be the main cause of these conditions.

Doctors have no silver bullet to treat cancer, and even fewer options for PTSD, so it's up to you to become informed. Depression, anxiety, cognitive disorders, suicide, addictions, divorce, and violence in our society are often consequences of unrecognized PTSD, as Dr. Jamie eloquently reveals.

I found Dr. Jamie's book to be an excellent, eye-opening intro-duction to what causes PTSD. She also reveals that many other conditions are actually symptoms of PTSD, rather than separate conditions. And she introduces a simple solution that is accessible to everyone.

Speaking as a practitioner, author, and researcher for the past 55 years, I enjoyed reading her book and even have discovered a few new things.

We should thank Dr. Jamie for devoting her life to improving our mental, physical and spiritual health. Now more than ever, we really need Dr. Jamie's book.

— Professor Serge Jurasunas, N.D (Hom), M.D (hc)

Dr. Jamie Turndorf is an amazing professional. In this very useful, practical book, she demonstrates, based on serious scientific data, that PTSD is a plague that underlies most diseases. She points out that we must take charge of our own heath and save ourselves. No lie, just love. Everyone seeks respect, but it starts with self-respect. Unfortunately, mainstream medicine does not try to cure people and instead creates addiction to chemical treatments. The nutritional aspect of life is still neglected, yet it is the core of good health. Stress is toxic to the brain, but most people think about using anxiolytic or illegal drugs to ease their symptoms. Hence, all these drugs create addictions and side effects without solving the problem. And these drugs create willing weakness. The loss of self-will makes it easier for government leaders to manipulate the people. But there are simple and safe solutions. This book shows you the way to identify your specific stress and break free of it. The real way out is to know yourself, to be yourself, and to participate actively in the rebuilding of your own health and dignity.

— Pascal Labouret, D.C. Hyeres, France

"This is an important and timely book that will only become more so as we move forward into even deeper chaos and economic decline. Dr. Turndorf insightfully alerts the world to the most important solution: heavy magnesium treatments through oral and transdermal approaches. She nails it on the head with magnesium, for it is the neurological mineral that calms us down. It is indicated for depression, for those on suicide watch, anxiety, and PTSD. One cannot go wrong with magnesium. Just be sure to take enough of it to get the best results."

-- Dr. Marc Sircus, author of Transdermal Magnesium Therapy

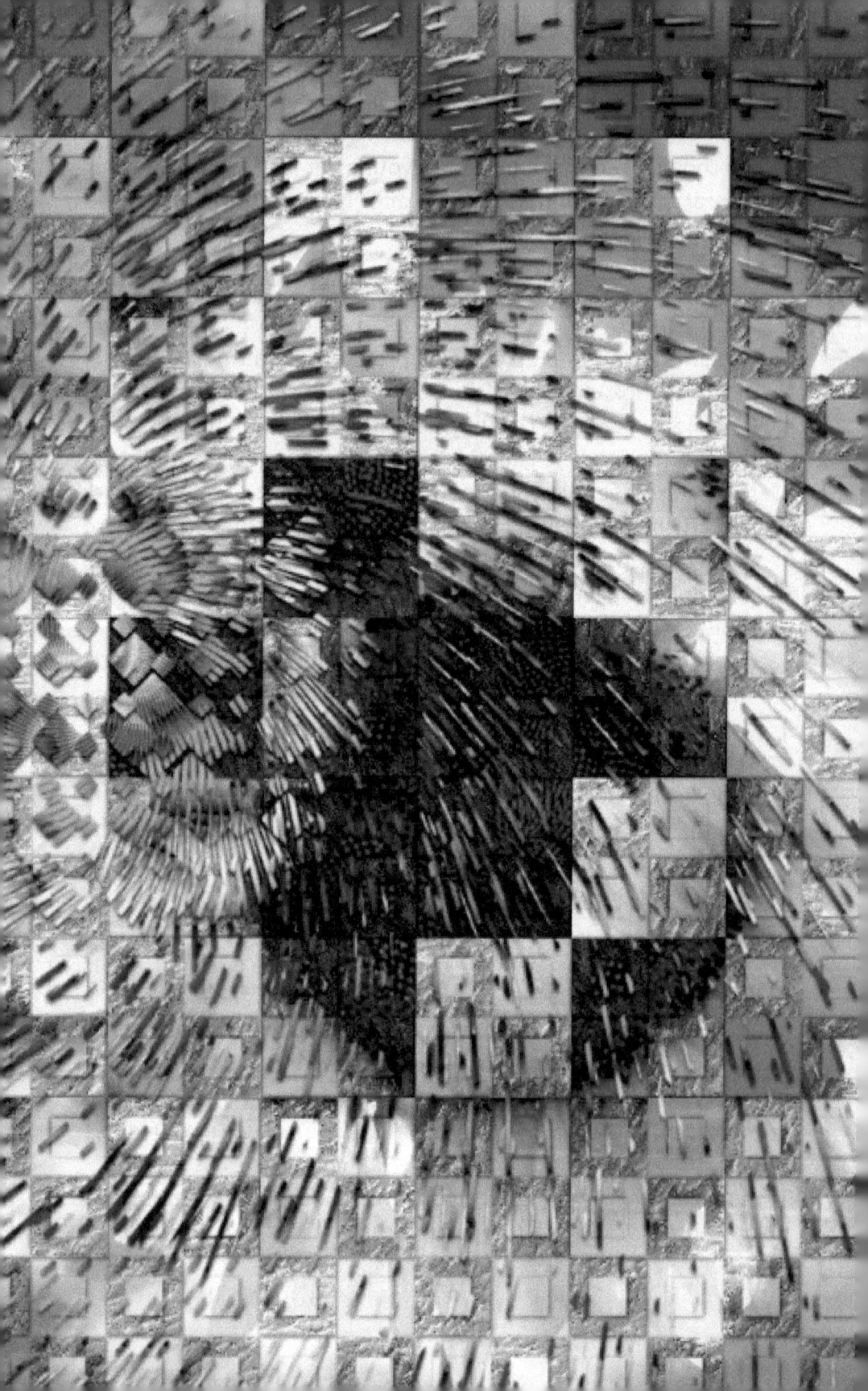

Contents

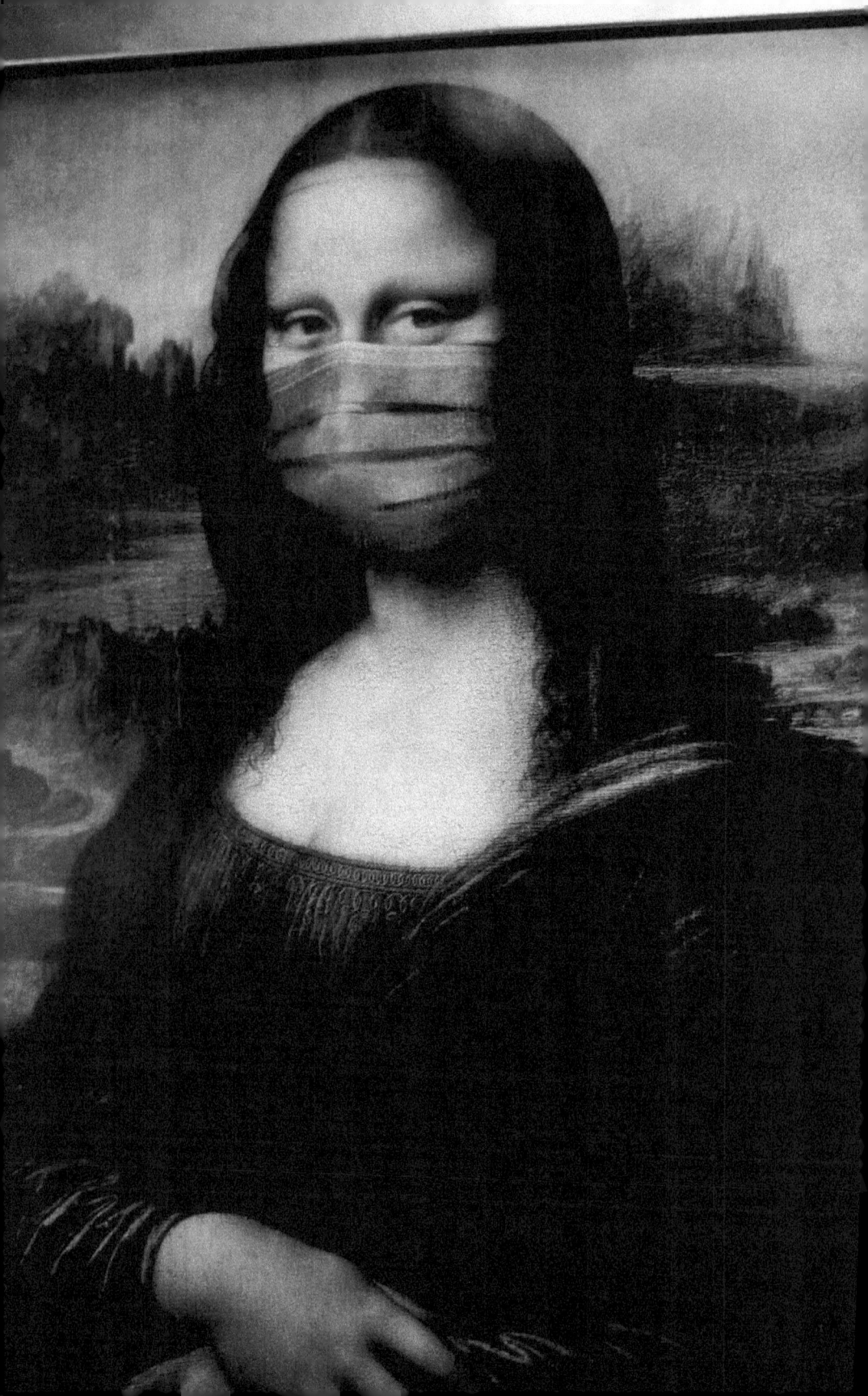

Preface

Are your nerves on edge?

Do you feel stressed-out, tense, anxious, jumpy or jittery?

Is your body stiff, sore, aching or painful?

Are you troubled by frightening thoughts that you or a loved one will die?

Is your mind overwhelmed with worry?

Do you have panic-attacks?

Or a racing or irregular heartbeat?

Are you feeling down and depressed or suffer debilitating, hopeless feelings like the world is coming to an end...or a sense of despondency (who cares if I eat right or exercise, the world is f***d)?

Are you avoiding doing what you know you should (like exercising or eating correctly)?

Do you sleep too much or have trouble sleeping?

Do you have nightmares?

Do you suffer flashbacks of previous traumas?

Do you avoid people and places that you know will upset you?

Are you engaged in self-damaging or addictive behaviors (such as bingeing on junk food) or self-medicating with drugs, alcohol or trapped in other addictive behaviors (such as online porn or binge Internet or TV viewing)?

If any of the above sounds like you, you could likely have PTSD.

Believe me, you're not alone.

According to the NIH (National Institute of Health), 44 million Americans including 5.5-6 million veterans reported struggling with PTSD as of June 2019. That statistic is the tip of the iceberg because most people don't even know they have PTSD and, therefore, don't receive treatment.

Here's a brief scientific breakdown of how PTSD happens to each of us. Read carefully, because even your doctor is likely not up on the latest research.

Stress (emotional, biochemical and/or environmental) causes a rapid and massive depletion of magnesium from the body.[1]

Magnesium loss triggers a chemical imbalance called HPA-Axis hypothalamic/pituitary/adrenal) dysfunction.[2]

The HPA-Axis refers to the primary neuro-biochemical stress response network that involves both the central nervous and endocrine systems. HPA-Axis dysfunction, hippocampal volume, and endogenous opioid function are technical terms that describe total adrenal burnout. Burnout is the end result of the body being trapped too long in fight-flight mode--also known as sympathetic arousal. Interestingly, for the last three decades, my own research has focused on developing effective communication and interactional techniques to abort this biochemical mechanism, which is triggered by unresolved relationship conflicts. Couples in conflict get stuck in a permanent state of chemical imbalance or chronic fight-flight mode, which is the same mechanism that occurs in PTSD.

HPA-Axis dysfunction is THE cause of PTSD*[3]

*Our poor Western diet and lifestyle, which includes impure water, processed foods, refined sugar and carbs, GMOs, gluten, damaged fats/oils**, fluoride toxicity and other neurotoxins and endotoxins, pharmaceutical drugs, toxic metals such as mercury, lead and aluminum, pesticides, and herbicides such as glyphosate residues in our food and water result in nearly every person being deficient in magnesium--meaning everyone has some degree of PTSDs.

Magnesium deficiency worsens with age, which explains why humans become sicker, less stress tolerant and more and more prone to PTSD as we grow older.

Don't despair. There is a way out.

In this book, I share a cutting-edge PTSD solution that your doctor also likely doesn't yet know about.

The good news is that the very same cause of PTSD and other stress related illnesses is the source of the solution! In short, according to much published NIH research, magnesium supplementation reverses PTSD.[4]

Unfortunately, in many cases oral magnesium causes diarrhea and gastrointestinal symptoms at worst, and 30% absorption, at best.[5]

This is why transdermal magnesium is preferable to oral magnesium for numerous reasons: it is more bioavailable and provides superior cellular absorption as it bypasses digestion and enters the bloodstream immediately to begin alleviating PTSD 6 and, as an additional bonus, transdermal magnesium moisturizes the skin.

If you're thinking, I'm not a veteran or a victim of abuse so I can't have PTSD, think again. All it takes is one single accident, illness or stressful event for the body to lose its magnesium stores and trigger PTSD.

As a result, we must all now face the painful truth: The stress associated with the Coronavirus pandemic (COVID-19) has pushed our magnesium deficient world over the edge, triggering what I have termed the *Global PTSD Pandemic Stress Syndrome*.

I am not telling you these dire statistics so that you will feel overwhelmed and develop a worse case of PTSD! That's the last thing you need! I'm telling you this because there are better drug-free options.

In the past year, I have been assisting people with the *Global PTSD Pandemic Stress Syndrome* using my *Energetic System Upgrade*™, a research-backed, divinely-inspired method (no, this method doesn't involve religion!) that produces amazingly transformational results.

How the *Energetic System Upgrade*™ Was Born

For nearly 30 years I was married to Emile Jean Pin, a world-renowned former Jesuit priest, Vatican professor, and founder of the Liberation Theology movement created to fight Church oppression from within. The Dalai Lama named him posthumously as one of the 50 men of all time who was one with God.

Fifteen years ago, my beloved Jean was mortally wounded by a bee while we were vacationing together in Italy.

Jean made his presence known to me the moment he left his body, proving to me, the former atheist, that we don't die! This realization led me to conclude that our relationships are not meant to end with "bodily" death; and, that we are meant to reconnect and stay connected, which is the only real cure for grief.

Having spent my entire professional career researching methods for resolving relationship conflict and fighting, I know that millions of people are not fortunate enough to have the chance to resolve issues before those close to us leave their bodies. As a result, most of us harbor unfinished business with someone in spirit.

Knowing that Western grief therapy methods offer us no way of healing unfinished business with those in spirit, combined with my realization that relationships are not meant to end with bodily death, inspired me to bring my Conflict-Resolution method to the world of after-death communication. This culminated in the creation of the *Trans-Dimensional Grief Resolution Method*. The cornerstone of my method is the *Dialoguing with the Departed* technique that guides the bereaved to reconnect and speak directly with those in spirit, enabling them to heal unfinished business.

I tell my amazing reconnection story and introduce the *Trans-Dimensional Grief Resolution Method* in my number 1 bestselling Hay House book, *Love Never Dies: How to Reconnect and Make Peace with the Deceased*.

One thing I never shared in *Love Never Dies* was a remarkable visitation from Jean right after he left his body.

I will never forget what happened. I was standing in the bedroom when Jean suddenly appeared to me and said, "I'm going to send you a man who is younger than you, never married, and who has no children." He added that the man would be grateful to me for saving his life the way I saved Jean's.

I was flabbergasted by what Jean said.

Then, life overtook me and I forgot about his message…

Until eleven years later when Jean sent that very man!

I'll never forget that day either…A tidal wave of love as large as eternity overtook me the minute I laid eyes on the man Jean sent.

As I soon discovered, Jean orchestrated the meeting to fill me with unearthly love for this man in order to assign me the divine appointment of healing vets with PTSD. Because, as I soon discovered, this man I instantly loved was a four-time Afghanistan war vet with severe PTSD.

It is my love for him that motivated me to find a real cure for him and for every vet who is suffering unresolved PTSD.

Through a series of painful events, that man withdrew before I could heal him, and I was simultaneously evicted from where I was living in New York.

I was so heartbroken and allowed the emotional riptide of that ruptured relationship to propel me from New York to Florida.

In Florida, the only way I could think to mend my broken heart was to pour my heart into finding a cure for vets with PTSD, the way I couldn't help the man I loved.

As I continued my research into PTSD, I soon realized that my PTSD mission was much broader than I had originally realized. I discovered that not only vets, but the majority of the population suffers undiagnosed PTSD.

In the process of researching the topic, I discovered that I, myself, had PTSD, as a result of: being born three months early and weighing only two pounds at birth; suffering emotional and physical abuse in my first family; suffering 106 degree fevers for the first 10 years of my life (the result of a congenital defect associated with my early birth); living on antibiotics for the first

10 years to treat the fevers; having surgery at age 10 to correct the defect; surviving a car crash in which a drunk driver rear-ended me while I was parked in traffic on a bridge; surviving a 60 mph train crash that caused spinal damage; having undetected and untreated Lyme disease for most of my adult life; and, last but not least, having my husband torn from me, due to a fatal bee sting. Yes, I had PTSD! I say "had" because I applied the same method that I developed to heal those with PTSD to myself, with equally amazing results.

Meanwhile, in Florida, I began sensing that I was being asked to develop a new energetic healing method that would enhance and expand upon the *Trans-Dimensional Grief Resolution Method*.

One day, I asked Jean to give me the name of the new method.

That night, in my online *Trans-Dimensional Grief Resolution Method* coaches training group, we all heard a bell ring, immediately followed by a woman's voice that said, "Excuse me. Time for a System Upgrade." We were all speechless because the voice didn't emanate from anyone's computer!

Now I had the name of the new method: The *Energetic System Upgrade*™!

But I still had no clue what this new method entailed and how it would relate to PTSD.

Around this time, I met the US distributors of a special form of magnesium called *Elektra Magnesium*. What's unique about this form of magnesium is that it's applied transdermally (via the skin). Because transdermal magnesium bypasses digestion and immediately enters the bloodstream, this form of magnesium has the power to instantly alleviate stress and PTSD! (Recall the research I cited above in which I said that stress excretes magnesium from the body and triggers PTSD, and supplementing with magnesium reverses PTSD.)

When I discovered **Elektra Magnesium**, the synchronicities that led me to this point hit me like a lightning bolt. I was moved to Florida as part of a divinely orchestrated plan to incorporate the **Elektra** transdermal magnesium as the first-step in my **Energetic System Upgrades™**. By the way, I don't sell the product. I'm not a distributor or affiliate.

In the past year, I've been using this special form of magnesium myself, and I prescribe it to my patients, and use it in my **Energetic System Upgrade™** live and online workshops with amazingly healing results not only with **Global PTSD Pandemic Stress Syndrome**, anxiety, panic and depression, but also in lifting any emotional, physical or spiritual blocks that most of us suffer.

As an aside, world-renowned Dr. Sherri Tenpenny just experienced her own healing miracle thanks to the **Energetic System Upgrade™**. She offered an unsolicited video testimonial in which she said that in just one session she experienced an 80% improvement of an issue that has plagued her for 45 years (and none of her previous healing efforts had made a dent in the issue).

How did I help her realize this shift? In short, all of us have suffered trauma in childhood, hence why I call childhood the "deformative" years! Trauma causes PTSD in all of us. Trauma has tentacles that reach into our adult lives and create painful blocks that interfere with our work life and/or interfere with our capacity to love and form satisfying intimate relationships. Early trauma is always working behind the scenes, on an unconscious level, and this makes us blind to the fact that an old trauma is causing our current discontent.

When I perform the **Energetic System Upgrade™**, I combine my skills as a psychoanalyst with my psychic abilities; the combination enables me to laser in and see the trauma that's causing your emotional, physical, relationship, work or spiritual block. When I make this link, it magically releases the tentacles that are taking hold of your life and causing your current pain, and this unlocks the block. That's why Dr. Tenpenny had such rapid improvement, because I uncovered the trauma that had its teeth in her, the trauma that had caused her lifelong issue. I want the same miracle for you.

As the first-step in my *Upgrades,* I use *Elektra Magnesium* because it instantly enters the bloodstream and begins reversing the chemical imbalance that underlies PTSD. As soon as the magnesium is applied to the skin, I literally see stress and PTSD vaporizing right in front of my eyes! My patients, workshop and webinar participants instantly feel calm but alert and receptive as the magnesium activates the electrical circuits in their brain, heart and organs. In this relaxed but open state, I then perform the *Energetic System Upgrade* in which I uncover and then uproot whatever underlying physical, emotional or spiritual imbalance, wound, trauma or unfinished business my patient or workshop participant is carrying. Healing the underlying emotional, physical and spiritual imbalances that underlie PTSD is vital because these factors are what set us up to fall prey to stress and PTSD in the first place; eliminating these underlying issues helps to ensure that PTSD doesn't return no matter how much stress one faces in the future.

*Magnesium and the good fats work together to create healthy cell wall function, which protects the cell contents, lets out wastes, and lets in water, glucose and insulin for proper metabolism. Magnesium also regulates the control of the calcium channels in the cell wall. When magnesium gets too low, the cell wall becomes leaky and compromised. A lot of this research about how stress depletes magnesium (via compromise of integrity of the cell membrane) was done and published by Mildred Seeling, who says:

"Auto-oxidation of catecholamines yields free radicals, which explains the enhancement of the protective effect of Mg by anti-oxidant nutrients against cardiac damage caused by beta-cat-echolamines. Thus, stress, whether physical (i.e. exertion, heat, cold, trauma--accidental or surgical, burns), or emotional (i.e. pain, anxiety, excitement or depression) and dyspnea as in asthma increases need for Mg."[7]

** In PTSD, the protective mechanism of cell membrane regulation is disturbed from stress, low magnesium and/or cellular acidity, which can cause a hyper-stimulation effect (too much glutamate and cortisol release), leaky gut, upset microbiome (from the acids), and anxiety. When we lose the integrity of our "nervous system insulation," when magnesium gets too low, our cholesterol fats become saturated with acids and then oxidize. This disturbed cell membrane regulation is the trigger that disrupts HPA-Axis function. As a consequence, we become hyper-sensitive, since we've lost our insulation or buffering capacities as the endocan-nabinoid nervous system becomes too raw. Good oils (unrefined omega 3 EFA oils), in conjunction with magnesium, work syner-gistically to calm, heal and seal the rawness and inflammation. According to Sandy Sanderson, magnesium researcher and creator of *Elektra Magnesium*, "The mechanism of action revolves around the connection of magnesium ions and how cholesterol (fats) works in the body. Fats/lipids perform insulating functions and also channel or funnel electron transfer in a controlled and balanced manner. We find the most cholesterol in the areas of highest electrical activity (50% in brain), and also in the structure of the nerve sheaths that insulate nerves. Lipids are present in the structure of the cell membrane itself as a phospholipid bilayer held together by magnesium ions. Lipids are integral in the epidermis for our skin barrier protection...Skin is also piezoelectric."

(Piezoelectric is relating to or involving electric polarization in a substance resulting from the application of mechanical stress.)

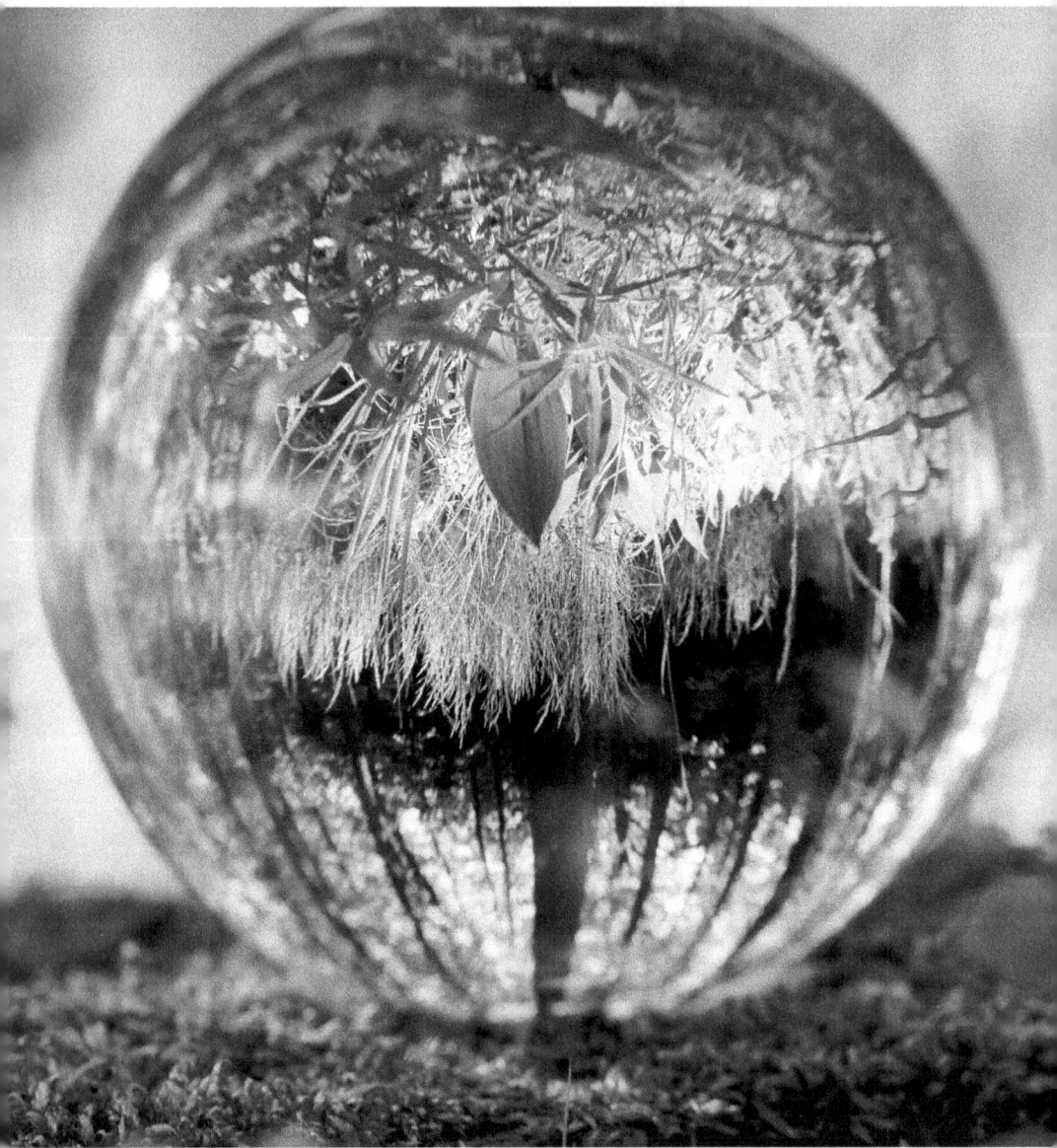

Introduction

PTSD as well as many other conditions and diseases are a magnesium deficiency in disguise.

I'll never forget the day that I had Carolyn Dean MD, the world's top magnesium expert, on my radio and TV show.

We discussed the fact that originally it was thought that magnesium is needed in 300 bodily functions, or enzyme systems to be precise, a number that was bumped up to 600. Dr. Dean and I also discussed the fact that the latest research shows magnesium is required in over 1000 enzyme systems.

Without adequate magnesium, humans fall prey to all kinds of diseases and conditions that are actually magnesium deficiency in disguise.

Here's a list of the diseases and conditions that are caused by magnesium deficiency. These same conditions can also be reversed with the use of magnesium.

1. Acid Reflux
2. Adrenal Fatigue
3. Alcoholism

4.   Allergies and Hay Fever

5.   Altitude Sickness

6.   Alzheimer's Disease

7.   Angina

8.   Anxiety and Panic Attacks

9.   Arthritis

10. Asthma

11. Atherosclerosis

12. Atrial Fibrillation/Arrythmia

13. Bipolar Disorder

14. Blood Clots

15. Blood sugar imbalances

16. Boils

17. Bowel Disease

18. Brain swelling

19. Bruxism (teeth grinding)

20. Cancer prevention

21. Carbuncles

22. Chemotherapy side effects

23. Cluster headaches

24. Cirrhosis

25. Confusion

26. Cystic Fibrosis

27. Calcification

28. Cardiac arrest

29. Cerebral Palsy

30. Cholesterol (lowering LDL (bad) cholesterol, raising HDL cholesterol)

31. Chronic Fatigue Syndrome (CFS)

32. Complex Regional Pain Syndrome

33. Constipation

34. Cystitis

35. Dementia
36. Depression
37. Detoxification
38. Diabetes (syndrome X, hyperinsulinemia, metabolic syndrome)
39. Epilepsy
40. Fatigue
41. Headaches
42. Head Trauma and Bleeding
43. Hearing Loss
44. Heart Disease
45. Hypertension (high blood pressure)
46. Hypoglycemia
47. Infection
48. Inflammation
49. Insomnia
50. Interstitial Cystitis
51. Irritable Bowel Syndrome (IBS)
52. Jellyfish Stings
53. Kidney Disease
54. Kidney Stones
55. Lyme Disease
56. Male Infertility
57. Mania
58. Memory problems
59. Migraine
60. Multiple Sclerosis
61. Musculoskeletal complaints
62. Muscle cramps
63. Fibrositis
64. Fibromyalgia
65. GI spasms
66. Tension headaches

67. Jaw spasms (TMJ)
68. Chronic neck and upper back pain
69. Low back pain
70. Neurological Manifestations
71. Trigeminal neuralgia
72. Muscle weakness
73. Skin sensitivity: tingling, twitching, tics, crawling, creeping, itching, prickling, numbness, pin, needles, stabbing, shocking, burning pain
74. Restless legs
75. Seizures and convulsions
76. Vertigo
77. Hyper-emotionality
78. Obstetrics/Gynecology
79. Premenstrual Syndrome (PMS)
80. Dysmenorrhea
81. Female infertility
82. Premature labor
83. Preeclampsia and Eclampsia
84. PTSD
85. Palpitations (heart)
86. Pancreatic infections
87. Parkinson's Disease
88. Osteoporosis
89. Poisoning
90. Raynaud's Syndrome
91. Sickle Cell Disease
92. Skin infections
93. Skin ulcers
94. Sudden Infant Death Syndrome (SIDS)
95. Sports Injuries
96. Sports Recovery
97. Strep bacteria

98. Temporomandibular Joint Syndrome (TMJ)
99. Tetanus
100. Tongue biting
101. Tooth decay
102. Urinary Incontinence
103. Wound healing problems

(Note that many of the above conditions are listed in Dr. Dean's book *The Magnesium Miracle*.8 My own research uncovered additional diseases and conditions that are not mentioned in Dr. Dean's book. Here is one source that cites most of the remaining diseases and conditions listed above.[9]

After Dr. Dean finished detailing her list of the 65 diseases and conditions named in her book, I noticed that she hadn't mentioned PTSD. I pointed this out to her and she was shocked. She, herself, hadn't made the connection between low magnesium and PTSD! She thanked me on-air for pointing out to her the unequivocal science linking low magnesium as the major factor in PTSD, and for also pointing out that supplementation with magnesium is a little-known PTSD remedy. If Dr. Dean, the world's expert on magnesium, hadn't known about the link between low magnesium and PTSD, you can be sure your MD is altogether unaware of this vital research.

As I was reminded again, there's always a silver lining to every sorrow. Had Jean not filled me with so much love for that vet with PTSD, I would never have been motivated to dig under every research rock to come up with the little-known PTSD and magnesium research.

Most people think, as I used to, that you can't have PTSD unless you're a veteran or someone who has suffered extreme violence or abuse. Not true. As I said in the foreword, all it takes is one stress, accident or illness to deplete our magnesium stores and trigger PTSD.

Most of us have suffered a degree of PTSD since childhood—who escapes childhood without an accident, illness or stress. Then we spend our lives trying to blot out symptoms with drugs, which further deplete our magnesium stores, making us sicker and sicker, and worsening PTSD.

As I said previously, the cumulative stress of life over time, combined with impure water, processed foods, refined sugar and carbs, alcohol, soda, certain foods such as tannins from black and green tea, phytic acid from unfermented soy products and unsoaked grains and seeds, oxalic acid from raw spinach, coffee, smoking, GMOs, gluten, damaged fats/oils, fluoride toxicity and other neurotoxins and endotoxins, pharmaceutical drugs (especially diuretics, bronchodilators such as theophylline for asthma, birth control pills, insulin, beta blockers, digitalis, tetracycline and some other antibiotics, corticosteroids, antipsychotics and cocaine) toxic metals such as mercury, lead and aluminum, pesticides and herbicides such as glyphosate residues in our food and water results in our becoming more and more depleted of magnesium. As magnesium levels lower over time, we all find ourselves teetering on the brink of PTSD (if we don't already have it). The stress of this latest viral pandemic is all that was required to push our magnesium deficient world over the edge, triggering what I now refer to as the *Global PTSD Pandemic Stress Syndrome*.

This book begins with an overview of PTSD symptoms, and a test to help you determine if you or someone you love is suffering from PTSD. Next, we will discuss how PTSD manifests differently in men versus women, followed by an overview of how PTSD expresses itself in children. Next, I take a close look at the symptom clusters associated with PTSD, grouping the main symptoms of

PTSD into four categories: 1) anxiety and panic, and their various emotional, physical and behavioral offshoots; 2) depressed mood and its emotional, physical and behavioral expressions; 3) pain syndromes; 4) PTSD and addiction; 5) next, I present how PTSD disrupts sexual functioning; and 6) lastly, we look at how the worldwide digestive disorders epidemic is actually a symptom of PTSD.

As you will soon discover, the symptoms associated with PTSD are themselves symptoms of low magnesium. And, again, correcting magnesium levels reverses PTSD and all its plaguing symptoms.

I close this chapter by entreating you to join forces with me to ensure that no body is left on the battlefield of PTSD.

Together we can become collective pebbles in the proverbial pond of love.

Together we can make the world a PTSD-free place.

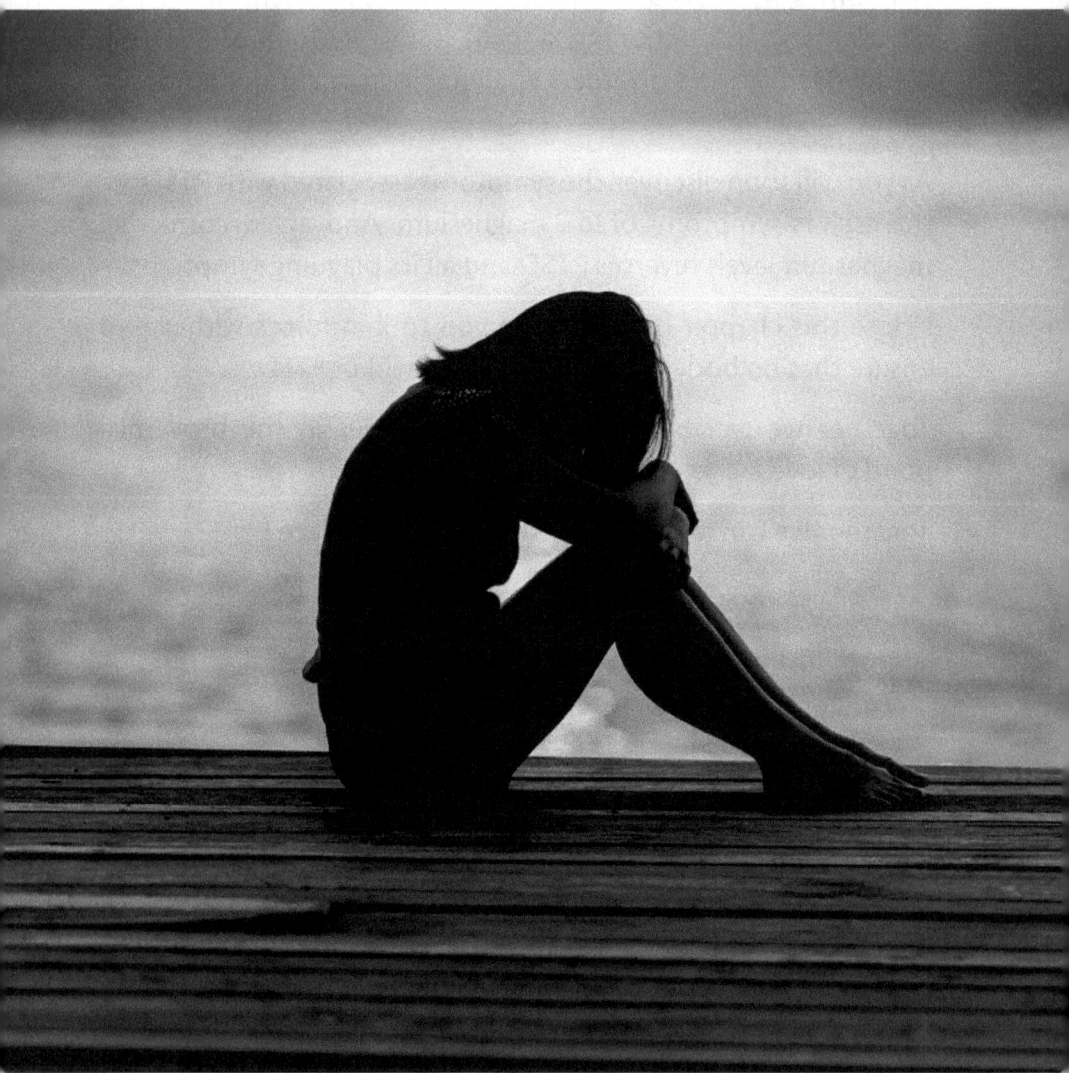

CHAPTER ONE
Could You or Someone You Love Be Suffering PTSD?

Life in Mary's first family was an emotional minefield. Her parents were always screaming at her and punishing her. Mary tried to be a good kid, she did, but she could never seem to figure out the rules of engagement. She was always in trouble for one offense or another, despite walking on eggshells to avoid setting off another emotional landmine.

Inevitably, she would commit yet another infraction and the "f" bombs would fly.

When her parents tired of yelling at her, she was sent off to solitary confinement in her room. Throughout her life, Mary has struggled with insomnia, irritability and headaches...

Keith was a clumsy kid. He was always tripping and falling off his bike. One day, he fell out of tree and broke his arm. From this point on, he never felt right in his skin. Throughout his life he's been sickly, nervous and forgetful...

According to the National Center for PTSD, about 6 of every

10 men (or 60%) and 5 of every 10 women (or 50%) experience at least one trauma in their lives. Women are more likely to experience sexual assault and child sexual abuse. Men are more likely to experience accidents, physical assault, combat, disaster, or to witness death or injury.[10]

When most of us think about PTSD, we imagine soldiers returning from the battlefield. Despite being a doctor, I initially felt called to the mission to cure veterans with PTSD because, like most of the world, I wrongly thought of PTSD as predominantly affecting vets!

But, as I've said previously, military veterans of wars on foreign shores are not the only PTSD sufferers.

Consider the above statistics: Sixty percent of men and fifty percent of women have experienced at least one trauma in their lifetimes.

The reality is PTSD is way more common than we think.

Millions of non-veterans silently struggle with PTSD suffered on the domestic battlefields of abusive family, marital and intimate relationships.

Domestic trauma takes many forms: Emotional or physical abuse or neglect during childhood, a divorce, a break-up, and even the bodily loss of a loved one.

And even if you manage to escape domestic drama and trauma, life also hurls illness and accidents upon you.

The reality is life is rife with a nearly infinite number of physical, emotional and spiritual stresses and traumas that are inevitable byproducts of our ride on the Earth plane.

And even if you were lucky enough to have a semi-functional family and escaped the various childhood accidents, illnesses and traumas that cause PTSD, the longer you live the more stresses you suffer. This means that the longer you live, the less likely you are to escape PTSD.

My point is, if you are living and breathing, you likely have a degree of PTSD!

How exactly do the physical, emotional and spiritual stresses and traumas of life cause PTSD?

As I stated previously, magnesium is excreted from the body in times of stress.

Magnesium depletion causes HPA-Axis dysfunction.[11]

HPA-Axis dysfunction causes PTSD.[12]

It's as simple as that.

It's important to remember that from the point of view of bio-chemistry, emotional, physical and spiritual stresses and traumas all create the same biochemical imbalance that triggers PTSD. In other words, the mind and body are truly one.

Here's another point. I'm sure you've heard the saying, "What doesn't get better, gets worse." In this context, I mean that magnesium depletion worsens as time goes on, which means that undiagnosed, untreated PTSD worsens as time goes by.

The question is how can you tell if you or someone you love has PTSD?

Let's examine the array of symptoms associated with PTSD.

According to the Anxiety and Depression Association of America, PTSD is diagnosed if a person suffers symptoms for at least one month following a traumatic event.

Keep in mind, symptoms may not appear for several months or even years following the trauma.

PTSD consists of three main types of symptoms:

- Re-experiencing the trauma through intrusive distressing recollections of the event, flashbacks, and nightmares.
- Emotional numbness and avoidance of places, people, and activities that are reminders of the trauma.
- Increased arousal such as difficulty sleeping and concentrating, feeling jumpy, and being easily irritated and angered.

Diagnostic criteria that apply to adults, adolescents, and children older than six include the following:

- Exposure to actual or threatened death, serious injury, or sexual violation.
- Directly experiencing the traumatic events.
- Witnessing, in person, the traumatic events.
- Learning that the traumatic events occurred to a close family member or close friend; cases of actual or threatened death must have been violent or accidental.
- Experiencing repeated or extreme exposure to aversive details of the traumatic events. (Examples are first responders collecting human remains; police officers repeatedly exposed to details of child abuse). Note: This does not apply to exposure through electronic media, television, movies, or pictures, unless exposure is work-related.

The presence of one or more of the following:

- Spontaneous or cued recurrent, involuntary, and intrusive distressing memories of the traumatic events. (Note: In children repetitive play may occur in which themes or aspects of the traumatic events are expressed.)
- Recurrent distressing dreams in which the content or affect (i.e. feeling) of the dream is related to the events. (Note: In children there may be frightening dreams without recognizable content.)
- Flashbacks or other dissociative reactions in which the

individual feels or acts as if the traumatic events are recurring. (Note: In children trauma-specific reenactment may occur in play.)

- Intense or prolonged psychological distress at exposure to internal or external cues that symbolize or resemble an aspect of the traumatic events.
- Physiological reactions to reminders of the traumatic events.

Persistent avoidance of distressing memories, thoughts, or feelings about or closely associated with the traumatic events or of external reminders (i.e., people, places, conversations, activities, objects, situations):

Two or more of the following:

- Inability to remember an important aspect of the traumatic events (not due to head injury, alcohol, or drugs).
- Persistent and exaggerated negative beliefs or expectations about oneself, others, or the world (e.g., "I am bad," "No one can be trusted," "The world is completely dangerous").
- Persistent, distorted blame of self or others about the cause or consequences of the traumatic events.
- Persistent fear, horror, anger, guilt, or shame.
- Markedly diminished interest or participation in significant activities.
- Feelings of detachment or estrangement from others.
- Persistent inability to experience positive emotions.

Two or more of the following marked changes in arousal and reactivity:

- Irritable or aggressive behavior
- Reckless or self-destructive behavior
- Hypervigilance
- Exaggerated startle response
- Problems with concentration

- Difficulty falling or staying asleep or restless sleep[13]

Take my PTSD Test

If after reading the above symptoms of PTSD, you suspect that you or someone you love is suffering from PTSD, I invite you to take my PTSD test. If you're answering on behalf of someone else, answer as accurately as possible.

On a scale of zero (being no/not an issue/not applicable) to 10 (being yes, highest) please answer the next questions honestly:

1. 1. I feel cut off/detached from others. 0, 1, 2, 3, 4, 5, 6, 7, 8, 9, 10
2. 2. I avoid going to places that bring up upsetting feelings or memories. 0, 1, 2, 3, 4, 5, 6, 7, 8, 9, 10
3. 3. I have been sexually assaulted. 0, 1, 2, 3, 4, 5, 6, 7, 8, 9, 10
4. 4. I blame myself for the assault I suffered. 0, 1, 2, 3, 4, 5, 6, 7, 8, 9, 10
5. 5. I was injured as a result of the assault I suffered. 0, 1, 2, 3, 4, 5, 6, 7, 8, 9, 10
6. 6. I have experienced a severe or life-threatening trauma. 0, 1, 2, 3, 4, 5, 6, 7, 8, 9, 10
7. 7. I had a severe reaction at the time of the trauma I suffered. 0, 1, 2, 3, 4, 5, 6, 7, 8, 9, 10
8. 8. I have experienced stressful events since the trauma. 0, 1, 2, 3, 4, 5, 6, 7, 8, 9, 10
9. 9. Sometimes I have strange physical reactions, such as rapid breathing, sweating, shaking or nausea when remembering or being reminded of past trauma. 0, 1, 2, 3, 4, 5, 6, 7, 8, 9, 10
10. 10. I do not have a good social support system. 0, 1, 2, 3, 4, 5, 6, 7, 8, 9, 10
11. 11. I need to be alone a lot. 0, 1, 2, 3, 4, 5, 6, 7, 8, 9, 10
12. 12. I feel a lot of stress and anxiety. 0, 1, 2, 3, 4, 5, 6, 7, 8, 9, 10
13. 13. I feel on edge/jittery/shaky/wired. 0, 1, 2, 3, 4, 5, 6, 7, 8, 9, 10

14.   14. If I were to be honest, I feel hopeless about the future. 0, 1, 2, 3, 4, 5, 6, 7, 8, 9, 10

15.   15. I feel I have nothing to live for. 0, 1, 2, 3, 4, 5, 6, 7, 8, 9, 10

16.   16. I have an irrational feeling that I'm going to die young. 0, 1, 2, 3, 4, 5, 6, 7, 8, 9, 10

17.   17. I feel sad and depressed. 0, 1, 2, 3, 4, 5, 6, 7, 8, 9, 10

18.   18. I engage in reckless behavior (e.g. driving too fast). 0, 1, 2, 3, 4, 5, 6, 7, 8, 9, 10

19.   19. I drink alcohol every day. 0, 1, 2, 3, 4, 5, 6, 7, 8, 9, 10

20.   20. I use street drugs, including marijuana. 0, 1, 2, 3, 4, 5, 6, 7, 8, 9, 10

21.   21. I have suicidal thoughts. 0, 1, 2, 3, 4, 5, 6, 7, 8, 9, 10

22.   22. I feel guilty to have survived my war buddies. 0, 1, 2, 3, 4, 5, 6, 7, 8, 9, 10

23.   23. I feel guilty over things I did in the war. 0, 1, 2, 3, 4, 5, 6, 7, 8, 9, 10

24.   24. I have attempted suicide. 0, 1, 2, 3, 4, 5, 6, 7, 8, 9, 10

25.   25. I often feel moody. 0, 1, 2, 3, 4, 5, 6, 7, 8, 9, 10

26.   26. I cry often. 0, 1, 2, 3, 4, 5, 6, 7, 8, 9, 10

27.   27. Noise or bright light bothers me. 0, 1, 2, 3, 4, 5, 6, 7, 8, 9, 10

28.   28. I am having problems in my relationships. 0, 1, 2, 3, 4, 5, 6, 7, 8, 9, 10

29.   29. I can't keep a relationship going. 0, 1, 2, 3, 4, 5, 6, 7, 8, 9, 10

30.   30. I often feel angry. 0, 1, 2, 3, 4, 5, 6, 7, 8, 9, 10

31.   31. I have angry outbursts. 0, 1, 2, 3, 4, 5, 6, 7, 8, 9, 10

32.   32. I am often irritable. 0, 1, 2, 3, 4, 5, 6, 7, 8, 9, 10

33.   33. I often feel confused. 0, 1, 2, 3, 4, 5, 6, 7, 8, 9, 10

34.   34. I have difficulty concentrating. 0, 1, 2, 3, 4, 5, 6, 7, 8, 9, 10

35.   35. I am often forgetful. 0, 1, 2, 3, 4, 5, 6, 7, 8, 9, 10

36.   36. I often feel overwhelmed. 0, 1, 2, 3, 4, 5, 6, 7, 8, 9, 10

37.   37. I am easily startled. 0, 1, 2, 3, 4, 5, 6, 7, 8, 9, 10

38.   38. I am overly alert, on guard/hyper-vigilant. 0, 1, 2, 3, 4, 5, 6, 7, 8, 9, 10

39.   39. I feel dizzy sometimes. 0, 1, 2, 3, 4, 5, 6, 7, 8, 9, 10

40.   40. I have flashbacks/intrusive memories. 0, 1, 2, 3, 4, 5, 6, 7, 8, 9, 10

41. 41. I avoid people or situations. 0, 1, 2, 3, 4, 5, 6, 7, 8, 9, 10
42. 42. I have problems with gambling. 0, 1, 2, 3, 4, 5, 6, 7, 8, 9, 10
43. 43. I am bothered by feelings of guilt. 0, 1, 2, 3, 4, 5, 6, 7, 8, 9, 10
44. 44. I have nightmares. 0, 1, 2, 3, 4, 5, 6, 7, 8, 9, 10
45. 45. I feel numb. 0, 1, 2, 3, 4, 5, 6, 7, 8, 9, 10
46. 46. I have a loss of interest or pleasure. 0, 1, 2, 3, 4, 5, 6, 7, 8, 9, 10
47. 47. I have a low sex drive. 0, 1, 2, 3, 4, 5, 6, 7, 8, 9, 10
48. 48. I numb myself with sexual activity—either masturbation or with a partner. 0, 1, 2, 3, 4, 5, 6, 7, 8, 9, 10
49. 49. I watch porn. 0, 1, 2, 3, 4, 5, 6, 7, 8, 9, 10
50. 50. My use of porn has been or is an issue in my relationships. 0, 1, 2, 3, 4, 5, 6, 7, 8, 9, 10
51. 51. I bury my pain in anonymous sex. 0, 1, 2, 3, 4, 5, 6, 7, 8, 9, 10
52. 52. I have been diagnosed with medical condition(s). 0, 1, 2, 3, 4, 5, 6, 7, 8, 9, 10
53. 53. I have been diagnosed with a mental health problem (like depression or anxiety). 0, 1, 2, 3, 4, 5, 6, 7, 8, 9, 10
54. 54. I take prescriptions medications recommended by my doctor. 0, 1, 2, 3, 4, 5, 6, 7, 8, 9, 10
55. 55. I take larger doses of my prescribed medication(s). 0, 1, 2, 3, 4, 5, 6, 7, 8, 9, 10
56. 56. I take prescription drugs without a doctor's script. 0, 1, 2, 3, 4, 5, 6, 7, 8, 9, 10
57. 57. I have hypertension (high blood pressure). 0, 1, 2, 3, 4, 5, 6, 7, 8, 9, 10. I don't know.
58. 58. I have low blood pressure. 0, 1, 2, 3, 4, 5, 6, 7, 8, 9, 10. I don't know.
59. 59. I have diabetes. 0, 1, 2, 3, 4, 5, 6, 7, 8, 9, 10. I don't know.
60. 60. I feel grumpy, irritable, jittery, shaky or get headaches when I don't eat. 0, 1, 2, 3, 4, 5, 6, 7, 8, 9, 10
61. 61. I have high cholesterol. 0, 1, 2, 3, 4, 5, 6, 7, 8, 9, 10. I don't know.
62. 62. I have hypothyroidism (low thyroid). 0, 1, 2, 3, 4, 5, 6, 7, 8, 9, 10. I don't know.

63. 63. I have hyperthyroidism (high thyroid). 0, 1, 2, 3, 4, 5, 6, 7, 8, 9, 10. I don't know.

64. 64. I am overweight. 0, 1, 2, 3, 4, 5, 6, 7, 8, 9, 10

65. 65. I carry excess weight around my stomach. 0, 1, 2, 3, 4, 5, 6, 7, 8, 9, 10

66. 66. I have cardiovascular disease or a heart rhythm disturbance. 0, 1, 2, 3, 4, 5, 6, 7, 8, 9, 10. I don't know.

67. 67. I suffer from muscle cramps, involuntary muscle movements or restless legs. 0, 1, 2, 3, 4, 5, 6, 7, 8, 9, 10

68. 68. I have skin problems like eczema, psoriasis or rashes. 0, 1, 2, 3, 4, 5, 6, 7, 8, 9, 10

69. 69. I have allergies. 0, 1, 2, 3, 4, 5, 6, 7, 8, 9, 10

70. 70. I have renal (kidney disorders). 0, 1, 2, 3, 4, 5, 6, 7, 8, 9, 10. I don't know.

71. 71. I have chronic fatigue, Lyme disease or fibromyalgia. 0, 1, 2, 3, 4, 5, 6, 7, 8, 9, 10

72. 72. I have or have had cancer. 0, 1, 2, 3, 4, 5, 6, 7, 8, 9, 10

73. 73. I have chronic pain, frequent headaches or arthritis (joint pain). 0, 1, 2, 3, 4, 5, 6, 7, 8, 9, 10

74. 74. I drink less than 2.5 liters of water per day. 0, 1, 2, 3, 4, 5, 6, 7, 8, 9, 10

75. 75. I eat processed/packaged foods or deep-fried foods. 0, 1, 2, 3, 4, 5, 6, 7, 8, 9, 10

76. 76. I have eating problems (eat too much, eat the wrong foods, or don't eat). 0, 1, 2, 3, 4, 5, 6, 7, 8, 9, 10

77. 77. I eat sugar or foods that contain high fructose corn syrup. 0, 1, 2, 3, 4, 5, 6, 7, 8, 9, 10

78. 78. I drink diet sodas. 0, 1, 2, 3, 4, 5, 6, 7, 8, 9, 10

79. 79. I have persistent digestive disorders such as heartburn/acid reflux, GERD, bloating, gut pain, leaky gut, constipation or diarrhea. 0, 1, 2, 3, 4, 5, 6, 7, 8, 9, 10

80. 80. I have a physical injury, which has caused permanent disability. 0, 1, 2, 3, 4, 5, 6, 7, 8, 9, 10

81. 81. I suffer chronic pain. 0, 1, 2, 3, 4, 5, 6, 7, 8, 9, 10

82. 82. I have trouble sleeping. 0, 1, 2, 3, 4, 5, 6, 7, 8, 9, 10
83. 83. I can't fall asleep. 0, 1, 2, 3, 4, 5, 6, 7, 8, 9, 10
84. 84. I can't stay asleep. 0, 1, 2, 3, 4, 5, 6, 7, 8, 9, 10

(FEMALES)

85. 85. I have irregular periods, excessive bleeding, endometriosis or excessive PMS symptoms. 0, 1, 2, 3, 4, 5, 6, 7, 8, 9, 10
86. 86. I am on the pill. 0, 1, 2, 3, 4, 5, 6, 7, 8, 9, 10

Scoring the Test

If you answered 6 or higher on more than four questions, you or someone you love is likely suffering PTSD.

I know that this discovery can be daunting, but hang in there!

As I've said previously, research proves that magnesium supplementation reverses PTSD. This means that there is a simple PTSD solution for you or someone you love as the following NIH published research proves. "Magnesium deficiency induces anxiety and HPA axis dysregulation: Modulation by therapeutic drug treatment"[14]

So, if the test revealed that you or someone you love likely suffers PTSD, please don't despair.

There is hope in sight, and by the time you finish reading this book, you (or someone you love) will already be well on your way to a PTSD-free life.

In the next chapter, we will focus on how PTSD manifests differently in men and women.

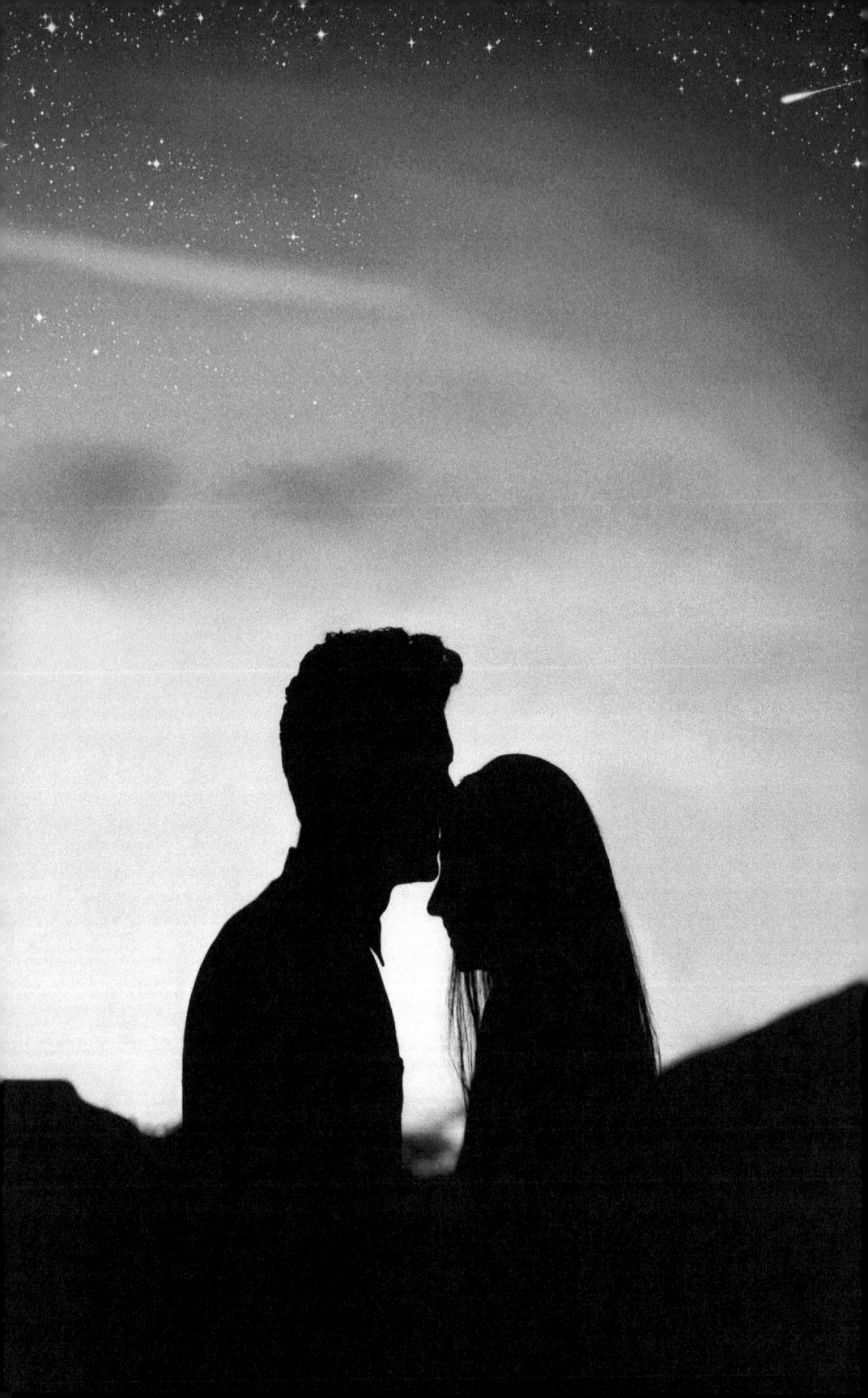

CHAPTER TWO
The Two Faces of PTSD: How PTSD Manifests Differently in Men Versus Women

In this chapter, we will examine the sex and gender differences in PTSD.

According to research, women are more than twice as likely to develop PTSD than men (12% for women and 6% for men).[15]

As I've previously stated, I believe the incidence of PTSD is much higher than we realize due to the fact that a single illness, accident or trauma depletes the body of magnesium. Magnesium depletion triggers hypothalamic/pituitary/adrenal (HPA-Axis) dysfunction. HPA-Axis dysfunction is the cause of PTSD.

Women are more prone to PTSD than men for several reasons:

High Impact Trauma

The first reason why women are more prone to PTSD is because women are exposed to more high-impact trauma. The higher the physical impact, the greater the risk of PTSD.

Of all forms of high impact assault, sexual assault is more likely to cause PTSD than any other event. One in four women (25%) are raped by age 44, as opposed to only 8% of men.

In addition, research shows that more women experience childhood neglect or abuse, and the sudden loss of a loved one, all of which are PTSD triggers.

Domestic violence is also a powerful PTSD trigger. According to the National Domestic Violence Hotline, each year over 12 million women and men are victims of intimate partner violence. Moreover, 35 percent of women worldwide have experienced either physical and/or sexual intimate partner violence or non-partner sexual violence, according to the United Nations.

Both men and women are at a higher risk of developing PTSD if they have a pre-existing mental health issue such as depression or anxiety, if their assault was severe, resulted in injury, and/or was life-threatening. If the reaction was extreme at the time of the assault, additional stress occurred after the trauma, and they do not have a good social support system, PTSD is likely to result.

The Earlier the Trauma the More Severe PTSD

Not only are women more likely to experience sexual assault, sexual abuse most commonly occurs at an earlier stage of life.

Trauma early in life has more impact in that it effects neurobio-logical, personality and brain development.

Initial Reaction to Trauma

Research shows that the stronger the initial reaction to a trauma, the greater risk of developing PTSD. Women generally score higher than men in terms of acute subjective responses, such as greater threat perception and dissociative reactions, which are known predictors of PTSD. A recent study compared physical and psychological reactions following a motor vehicle accident. The researchers studied initial heart rate and urinary cortisol levels along with emotional reactions such as initial perceived life threat. The research found that the severity of initial reaction to the trauma was linked to the severity of PTSD. According to this research, women's physical and psychological reactions to the trauma were stronger than men's reactions.[16]

Self-Blame and PTSD

Self-blame is also linked to a higher incidence of PTSD. Because women are more likely to be sexually assaulted, there is more self-blame associated with this kind of trauma. Therefore, women, as opposed to men, are more likely to blame themselves for their assault.

While men also experience traumas like sexual assault, abuse, and domestic violence, the occurrence rate is much lower.

For men, combat trauma is most associated with PTSD. However, combat trauma generally produces less shame and other negative feelings about oneself.

Different Physical Reactions to Trauma

Traumatic stress affects different areas of the brains of boys and girls at different ages.

Women have a two to three times higher risk of developing post-traumatic stress disorder (PTSD) compared to men. Several factors are involved explaining this difference:[17]

Stress responses activate the HPA-Axis in the brain. In individuals with PTSD, the HPA-Axis response is dysregulated, as I've stated repeatedly.

HPA-Axis dysfunction causes the release of the stress hormone cortisol. The more severe the trauma, the more cortisol released.

People with PTSD generally have lower amounts of cortisol circulating through their bodies—this may be due to end-stage adrenal fatigue—which ultimately results in low cortisol levels.

According to research, women appear to have a more sensitized hypothalamus/pituitary/adrenal (HPA-Axis) than men, while men appear to have a sensitized physiological hyperarousal system. PTSD has consistently been associated with amygdala hyperactivity, ventromedial prefrontal cortex (vmPFC) hypoactivity, and reduced communication (functional connectivity) between the vmPFC and amygdala, with the lower PFC control over the amygdala providing an explanation for the excessive fear response in PTSD.[18]

For those suffering PTSD, when a traumatic memory is recalled, memories don't fade over time as they do in people with normal-functioning HPA axis responses.

The HPA axis is more sensitive and responds more strongly to stress in females than males, especially during certain points in the menstrual cycle. If a woman is later in her cycle, her brain will release more cortisol.

Therefore, if a traumatic event happens to a woman while she is in the luteal phase of her menstrual cycle instead of follicular, she's more likely to develop flashback symptoms and PTSD.

Men are vulnerable to developing post-traumatic stress disorder in other ways. Specifically, the hippocampus—the part of the brain that forms memories—decreases in volume in men with PTSD.

The decrease is more pronounced in men than in women. This means that women with PTSD have less memory loss and cognitive impairment as a result of trauma than men do.

Men also appear to have a more sensitive hyperarousal system. This means they're more likely to experience symptoms like paranoia and impulsivity[19]

PTSD Symptoms in Men and Women

Men and women can and do experience the same PTSD symptoms. Nevertheless, specific symptoms are more common among women versus men and vice versa. For example, women are more likely to feel edgy, cut-off or detached from the feelings associated with the trauma, and they also tend to avoid things that remind them of the trauma.

Men tend to feel angry and experience angry outbursts more often than women. Women with PTSD are more likely to feel depressed and anxious, while men with PTSD are more likely to have problems with alcohol or drugs. Both women and men who experience PTSD may develop physical health problems.

PTSD Symptoms in Men Versus Women

Women are more likely to experience:

- Emotional numbness
- Avoidance symptoms
- Mood and anxiety disorders
- Shame and self-blame

Men are more likely to experience:

- Irritability
- Impulsivity

- Substance use disorders
- Paranoia
- Exaggerated startle response

Treatment Responses to PTSD

Gender-role differences play a role in PTSD treatment outcomes. First, women tend to seek social support and help more frequently than do men. And, women also tend to be more comfortable speaking about their emotions, which may explain why women have been shown to benefit more from psychotherapy in the treatment of PTSD.

Men more commonly resort to substance use to quell their PTSD symptoms. Angry outbursts are another common form of male "coping."

Research on treatments for PTSD do not focus on which treatments are more effective based on sex or gender.

Mainstream treatments include CBT (Cognitive-Behavioral Therapy), Drugs, EMDR (Eye Movement and Desensitization and Reprocessing) and, the new kid on the block: Transcranial Magnetic Stimulation (TMS). Research is unclear if TMS is effective in treating PTSD.[20]

Perhaps because none of the treatments to date have been particularly effective in resolving PTSD, another experimental treatment called Deep Brain Stimulation has appeared on the scene. This surgical procedure involves stimulation of the amygdala, ventral striatum, hippocampus, and prefrontal cortex.

The idea of this procedure is to surgically turn off the HPA-Axis dysfunction that has caused the brain and body of PTSD sufferers to get stuck in overdrive.

Why on earth would we subject PTSD sufferers to a risky surgical procedure and unknown effects of long-term neurostimulation when documented NIH research demonstrates that magnesium is a safe and natural central nervous system depressant that reverses HPA-Axis dysfunction and PTSD?[21,22]

Because oral administration of transdermal magnesium results in, at best, a 30% absorption rate, and because transdermal magnesium results in superior intracellular absorption, I believe transdermal magnesium is the surest and most effective remedy for those suffering PTSD.[23]

If you or someone you love is suffering PTSD, rather than subject yourself or them to minimally effective-at-best-and-risky-at-worst treatments, please make transdermal magnesium your first treatment option. In the next chapter, we will look at how PTSD manifests in children.

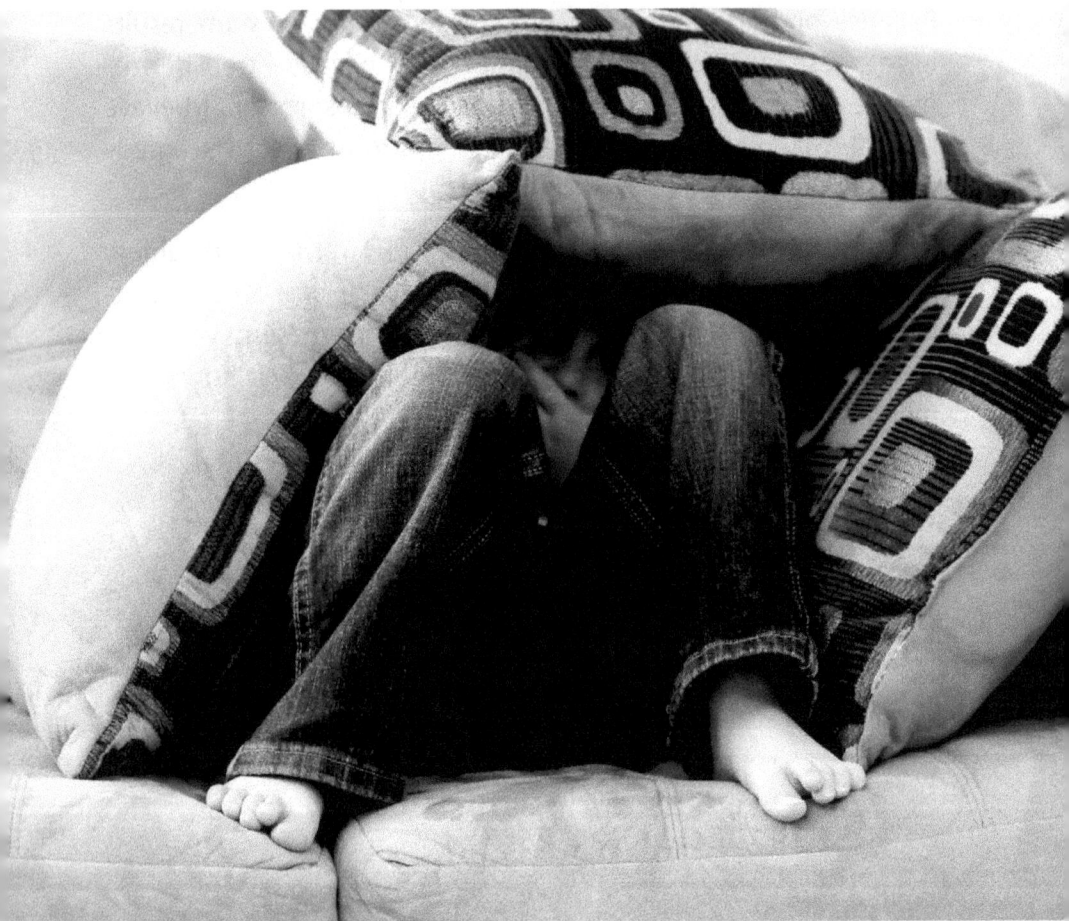

CHAPTER THREE
Recognizing PTSD in Our Children

According to the National Center for PTSD, about 15% to 43% of girls and 14% to 43% of boys experience at least one trauma in childhood.

Official statistics show that among children and teens who have experienced a trauma, 3% to 15% of girls and 1% to 6% of boys develop PTSD.

I argue that the incidence of PTSD among children and teens is much higher than we think.

Why do I say this?

Because:

Trauma depletes cellular magnesium levels.[24]

(To remind you, only one traumatic event is sufficient to deplete magnesium levels.)

And magnesium depletion triggers HPA-Axis dysfunction.[25]

Research proves that HPA-Axis dysfunction causes PTSD.[26]

Because we know that a single trauma is sufficient to set off the chemical cascade that results in PTSD, and because we know that almost 50% of all children and teens have experienced a trauma, it is, therefore, realistic to argue that nearly half of all boys and girls likely suffer some degree of PTSD.

What Events Cause PTSD in Children?

According to the National Center for PTSD, there are approximately three million child protection services annual reports involving 5.5 million children just in the US.

Of the reported cases, there is proof of abuse in about 30%. Of the reported cases of abuse, 65% are attributed to neglect, 18% to physical abuse, 10% to sexual abuse, and 7% to psychological (mental) abuse.

When we think of PTSD in children or teens, we think of mass shootings, like the Parkland Florida shooting. Clearly, children who have suffered these kinds of traumas suffer extreme PTSD.

It's important to note that there are many other kinds of events that trigger PTSD.

Keep in mind that reactions to trauma differ from child to child. For example, if a child has a pre-existing mental health issue, takes pharmaceutical drugs, consumes a poor diet containing fast foods, packaged foods, refined sugars and sodas, high-fructose corn sweetener and unhealthy fats, that child will be nutritionally deficient in magnesium. In such cases, a small trauma can have catastrophic effects by flushing out the little magnesium that is available, thereby triggering PTSD.

In addition, if a child doesn't have a good support system, and, therefore, has no way of working through the emotional aspects of a trauma, PTSD is more likely to occur.

The following is a list of the kinds of events that are likely to trigger PTSD:

- Natural disasters like floods and hurricanes
- Family dysfunction (arguments, physical fights)
- Losing one's residence/frequent moves
- Surviving war or violent events like mass shootings
- Being the victim of bullying
- Death of a loved one
- Parental divorce or separation
- A friend's or relative's suicide
- Attacks from animals such as dog bites
- Neglect from a parent or caregiver
- Car accidents
- Fires
- Physical abuse
- Pressure to perform at school or in sports
- Illness
- Physical accidents or injury
- Sexual abuse
- Personal attacks such as robbery or rape
- Emotional abuse from family or peers
- Witnessing violence
- Witnessing a serious accident, injury or death
- Substance abuse
- Vaccinations

PTSD Symptoms in Children and Teens

According to the NIH, PTSD symptoms manifest differently in young children, school-age children, teens, and adults. In addition, every child's symptoms vary.

The following are guidelines of how PTSD manifests in children and teens:

PTSD Symptoms in Children

Because young children are pre-verbal, thoughts and feelings will be communicated through behaviors rather than words.

Young children (below 5)

- Reluctance to leave their parent or caregiver
- Shaking or trembling
- Becoming catatonic: sitting still or not speaking
- Wetting the bed
- Sucking their thumb
- Reverted behavioral development: acting like they're at a younger age
- New or unusual phobias such as fear of dark or small spaces

School-aged children (6-11)

- Aggressive behavior like fighting
- Isolating themselves or refusing to talk
- Developing irrational fears
- Losing interest in activities
- Unusually poor school work
- Feeling guilty for things that aren't their fault
- Complaining of nonexistent physical health problems

Adolescent PTSD Symptoms

Teens and preteens (12-17) aren't quite adults but they aren't children either. Depending on a teen's age and personality, he or she may express PTSD symptoms that either fall into the adult or child category. These may include:

- Flashbacks such as memories reliving the traumatic event
- Substance abuse
- Symptoms of depression such as isolating or losing interest in fun activities
- Symptoms of anxiety
- Increased aggression, irritability, or hostility
- Suicidal thoughts
- Self-destructive, disrespectful, or dangerous behaviors
- Avoiding places and people that remind them of the traumatic event
- Insomnia, nightmares, or sleep disturbances
- Expressing wishes for revenge
- Expressing guilt for not preventing the event[27]

How to Help Children and Teens Suffering PTSD

When I reviewed the prevailing mainstream treatments for children and teens with PTSD, I sadly discovered what I was afraid I would. Treatment recommendations include individual and group psychotherapy, relaxation training, revisiting the trauma narrative, EMDR, and psychotropic medications.

These recommendations are noticeably lacking the most vital element: magnesium.

I remind you: Trauma depletes magnesium, and magnesium depletion triggers HPA-Axis dysfunction and PTSD.

And, most importantly, research proves that magnesium supplementation reverses the bio-chemical imbalance that causes PTSD.[28]

Make no mistake. No amount of love, talking therapies and/or therapeutic techniques can reverse magnesium deficiency! This means that talking and other therapeutic techniques will only be marginally effective in healing PTSD—which is why research to date has always shown PTSD to be particularly intractable to treatment.

Not any longer!

It's well known that cutting-edge research often takes decades to permeate mainstream practice—and this includes magnesium research.

We cannot afford to wait until doctors and mental health practitioners discover the proven research demonstrating the power of magnesium to reverse PTSD.

I am asking you to join my magnesium mission: Spread the word that magnesium needs to be the first line of treatment for every child and teen who is suffering PTSD.

One more point: because oral magnesium supplementation results in, at best, 30% absorption, transdermal magnesium is the preferred delivery method.

It is my wish that, together, we can finally make huge inroads in healing the PTSD epidemic plaguing our children and teens.

Together we can ensure that every child and teen suffering PTSD finds relief.

Note: In addition to trauma-depleting magnesium levels, triggering HPA-Axis dysfunction and PTSD, it's important to note that children can be born with a magnesium deficiency if their parents were deficient. This is an epigenetic hand-me-down that can be corrected using high doses of magnesium, which can also change genetic expression.

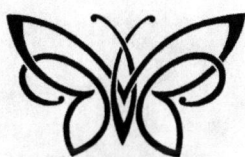

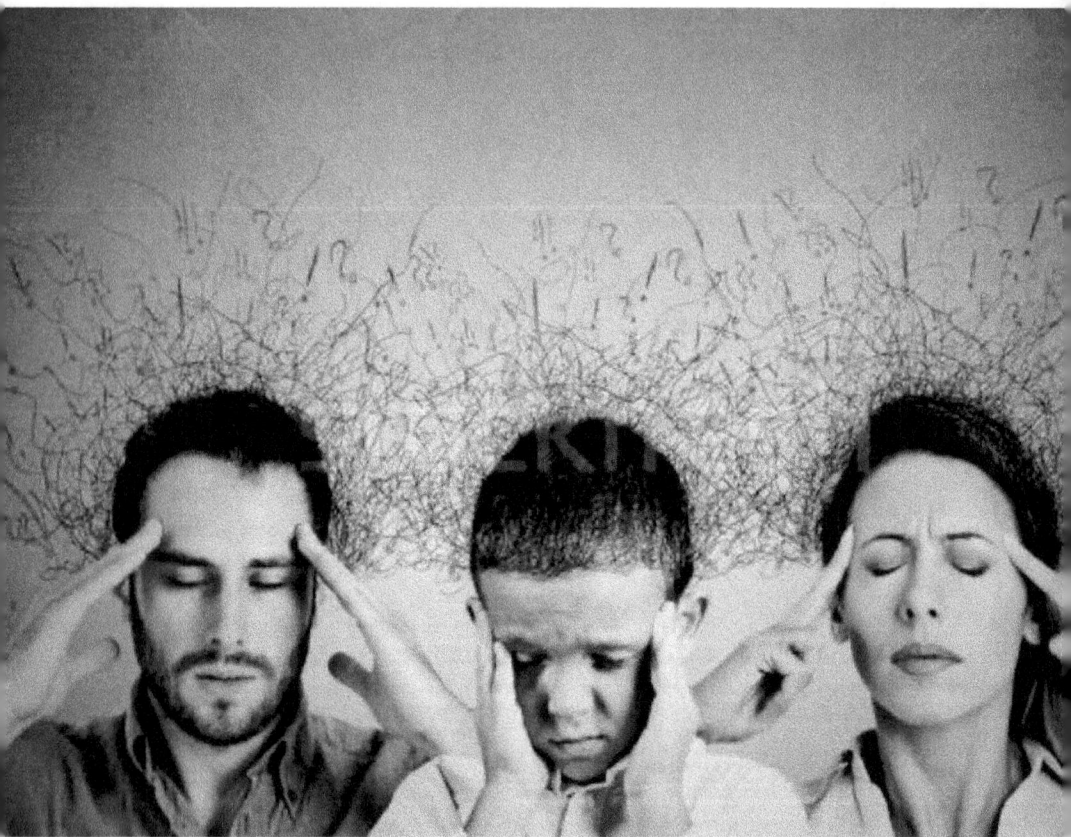

CHAPTER FOUR
Do you Have Panic, Anxiety or PTSD?

Do you feel easily tired, restless, jumpy and hypervigilant?

Do you have difficulty concentrating or sleeping, or suffer muscle tension, irritability and/or angry outbursts?

Do you experience nightmares or flashbacks of upsetting events?

Does your heart often race?

Do you suffer shortness of breath and facial flushing?

Do you avoid people, places or activities that you fear will trigger these upsetting physical reactions?

If you said yes to any of the above questions, you could be suffering from Generalized Anxiety Disorder (GAD), Panic Disorder or PTSD, or a combination of all three.

To complicate matters, one condition can predispose you to the other conditions. For example, if you are prone to anxiety, you are more at risk of developing PTSD.

The question is how can you know which condition(s) you're suffering from?

To answer that question, let's take a look at the similarities and differences of all three conditions.

The Anxiety and Depression Association of America states that Generalized Anxiety Disorder (GAD) affects 6.8 million people worldwide and 3.1 million in the US.

According to the Diagnostic and Statistical Manual of Mental Disorders, 5th edition, the hallmark of Generalized Anxiety Disorder is excessive worry and anxiety.

And at least 3 of the following 6 symptoms:

- Restlessness, feeling keyed up or on edge
- Being easily fatigued
- Difficulty concentrating or mind going blank
- Irritability
- Muscle tension
- Sleep disturbance (difficulty falling or staying asleep, or restless, unsatisfying sleep)

In addition, the above symptoms must occur more days than not for at least 6 months, and:

- Cause significant disturbance in social, occupational or other important areas of functioning
- Not be attributable to a medical condition (such as hyperthyroidism), or a physiological reaction to a drug
- The symptoms must also not be better explained by another condition, such as Social Anxiety Disorder, Separation Anxiety or Obsessive-Compulsive Disorder, or be secondary to the fear of having panic attacks, which is a common symptom of Panic Disorder
- Not be associated with reminders of traumatic events, as is the

case of PTSD, or fear of gaining weight, as in anorexia nervosa or Body Dysmorphic Disorder

• And not be associated with a serious illness, or related to delusions in schizophrenia

Now let's look at Panic Disorder.

Panic attacks are the central feature of Panic Disorder. The DSM-5 divides panic attacks into two categories: expected and unexpected panic attacks.

Expected panic attacks are linked to a specific fear, such as fear of heights. Unexpected panic attacks occur without any clear trigger, and seem to appear out of the blue.

According to the DSM-5, a panic attack is characterized by four or more of the following symptoms:

• Palpitations, pounding heart, or accelerated heart rate
• Sweating
• Trembling or shaking
• Sensations of shortness of breath or smothering
• A feeling of choking
• Chest pain or discomfort
• Nausea, vomiting or abdominal distress
• Feeling dizzy, unsteady, lightheaded, or faint
• Feelings of unreality (derealization) or being detached from oneself (depersonalization)
• Fear of losing control or going crazy
• Fear of dying
• Numbness or tingling sensations (paresthesias)
• Chills or hot flushes

A limited-symptom panic attack is diagnosed if less than four of the above symptoms are present.

What about Post-Traumatic Stress Disorder?

PTSD is considered a type of anxiety disorder that develops after experiencing or witnessing a traumatic event. The fearful feelings associated with PTSD overlap the feelings one experiences with Generalized Anxiety and Panic Disorders.

Symptoms of PTSD include many of the same symptoms we see in GAD and Panic Disorder, such as:

- Sleep pattern disturbances
- Irritability
- Angry outbursts
- Difficulty concentrating
- Emotional numbness
- Hypervigilance
- Feeling jumpy or easily startled

As you can see, the above psychological and physiological symptoms are identical to those of GAD and Panic Disorders.

The real difference between these other two disorders and PTSD is that it's common for PTSD sufferers to become triggered by events, places or objects, which results in a re-living of the original trauma through flashbacks, hallucinations and nightmares.

When triggered, the PTSD sufferer may develop a pattern of avoiding people and places that are associated with the trauma.

To confuse matters, avoidant behavior can be seen in those suffering GAD or Panic Disorders. However, those with GAD or Panic Disorders may avoid people or places at which anxiety or panic was previously experienced, causing the GAD or Panic Disorder sufferer to avoid specific places and situations for fear of triggering more anxiety or panic.

While many symptoms of GAD and Panic Disorder overlap, PTSD symptoms generally include the following:

- Resistance to talk about, think about or feel anything related to the trauma
- Avoiding places, activities and people that trigger memories of the trauma
- Difficulty recalling details about the event or events
- Avoiding activities that used to be enjoyable
- Feeling cut-off, isolated and detached from others
- Decreased interest in activities
- A feeling of numbness and a flatness of emotions
- Difficulty feeling positive feelings
- Overwhelming negative affect
- Believing that a normal future, life or lifespan is not possible
- Risky or destructive behavior
- Irritability or aggression
- Negative self-image, self-blame and guilt
- Heightened startle response
- Hypervigilence
- Difficulty concentrating
- Difficulty sleeping

Now that you have read the symptoms and diagnostic criteria for these three very similar conditions, let's talk about treatment options.

If you weren't scared before, you should be scared by what I will tell you next.

Over my 37 years as a clinician, I can't tell you how many horror stories I've witnessed that go something like the following:

A patient experiences anxiety, panic or intrusive PTSD symptoms such as fear, nightmares, flashbacks, insomnia, etc.

41

That patient visits his/her primary care physician or goes to the ER.

Mainstream docs tell that person that we don't really understand what causes these conditions, there is no cure, and that he/she should be prepared to spend the rest of his/her life "managing" the condition.

Mainstream medicine's way of "managing" these conditions is to prescribe pharmaceutical drugs, such as SSRIs and SNRIs in combination with anti-anxiety medication. (I frankly never understood why Western medicine takes such pains to establish differential diagnoses in order to assign the "right" label for a patient's psychiatric condition when the same class of drugs are used all the same!)

After beginning the medication, the patient may feel some relief, but drugs become less effective over time as the body adapts to them; and the patient's doctor will keep raising the dose. Eventually, the original symptoms bleed through all the same.

Sooner or later, the patient tries to discontinue the drugs.

Here's where true hell begins.

In attempting to get off these pharmaceutical drugs, the patient experiences worse symptoms than before starting the drug.

Western medicine has all kinds of names for drug withdrawal reactions: Discontinuation Syndrome, Withdrawal Phenomenon, or Rebound Phenomenon.

No matter what you call it, it's still hell.

There are actually rehab programs designed to address this problem.

And there are many published articles on this topic.[29]

I'll never forget a young psychotherapist who came to me for treatment to address her profound anxiety as a result of trying to get off her anti-anxiety medication. She was disabled with worse anxiety than before she began the drug.

As you can surely tell by now, I'm no fan of pharmaceutical drugs, which only treat symptoms and cause side effects that actually worsen the underlying cause of what ails us.

Until you uncover the underlying cause of your symptoms, it will be nearly impossible to overcome your anxiety, panic and PTSD.

What is the underlying cause of these three conditions?

Mainstream medicine will tell you that one or more of the following is to blame:

- Brain chemistry imbalances
- Hormone imbalance
- Genetic predisposition
- Low self-esteem
- Borderline personality disorder
- Physical or sexual abuse
- Chronic diseases like diabetes, multiple sclerosis and cancer
- Abuse of alcohol or drugs
- Certain prescription medications
- Family history of depression
- Age, gender, race and geography

Alternative medicine has other theories to explain anxiety, panic and PTSD disorders, which include:

- Blood sugar imbalances
- Mineral imbalances
- Thyroid disorders/diseases
- Hyperacidity

- Metal toxicity
- Adrenal fatigue
- Food allergies or sensitivities
- Chemical sensitivities and reactions caused by Leaky Gut/ Intestinal Permeability
- GMOs, herbicides (e.g. glyphosate), pesticides, and agriculture chemicals
- Liver toxicity and compromised detox ability
- Drug side effects
- A deficiency or imbalance of the Essential Fatty Acids (EFAs)
- A deficiency or imbalance of major and trace minerals

What if I told you there may well be a simple way to cut to the chase and address the underlying cause of your GAD, Panic Disorder and PTSD?

Transdermal Magnesium!

We know that magnesium is required in over 1,000 enzyme systems, including blood sugar regulation, heart rate and rhythm, central nervous system, and brain functions, all of which are integrally connected to mood. Magnesium is the eleventh most abundant element by mass in the human body and is essential to all cells and these 1,000 enzymes. Magnesium ions interact with polyphosphate compounds such as ATP, DNA, and RNA. Hundreds of enzymes require magnesium ions to function. Magnesium compounds are used medicinally as common laxatives, antacids (e.g., milk of magnesia), and to stabilize abnormal nerve excitation or blood vessel spasm in such conditions as eclampsia.

We also know that the majority of the population is deficient in magnesium.

And we know that oral magnesium is not always well-absorbed by everyone.

The bottom line is this:

If you are suffering any of the above conditions, your first line of treatment should be transdermal magnesium.

I have seen astounding improvements in patients suffering all forms of anxiety, panic and PTSD using transdermal magnesium.

Whereas drugs deplete the body of magnesium—which may explain why drugs ultimately worsen our health and cause us to develop worsening anxiety and panic, as well as new conditions—magnesium addresses the underlying cause of most every condition!

You have nothing to lose or risk and everything to gain in making magnesium your first line of treatment for GAD, Panic Disorder and PTSD.

Please note: If you are already taking pharmaceutical drugs, do not stop cold turkey. Only reduce the dose according to your doctor's schedule, while adding transdermal magnesium to your treatment regime. By treating the underlying magnesium deficiency, you should experience an easier withdrawal from the pharmaceutical drug and an overall improvement in the symptoms that led you to take the prescription drug in the first place.

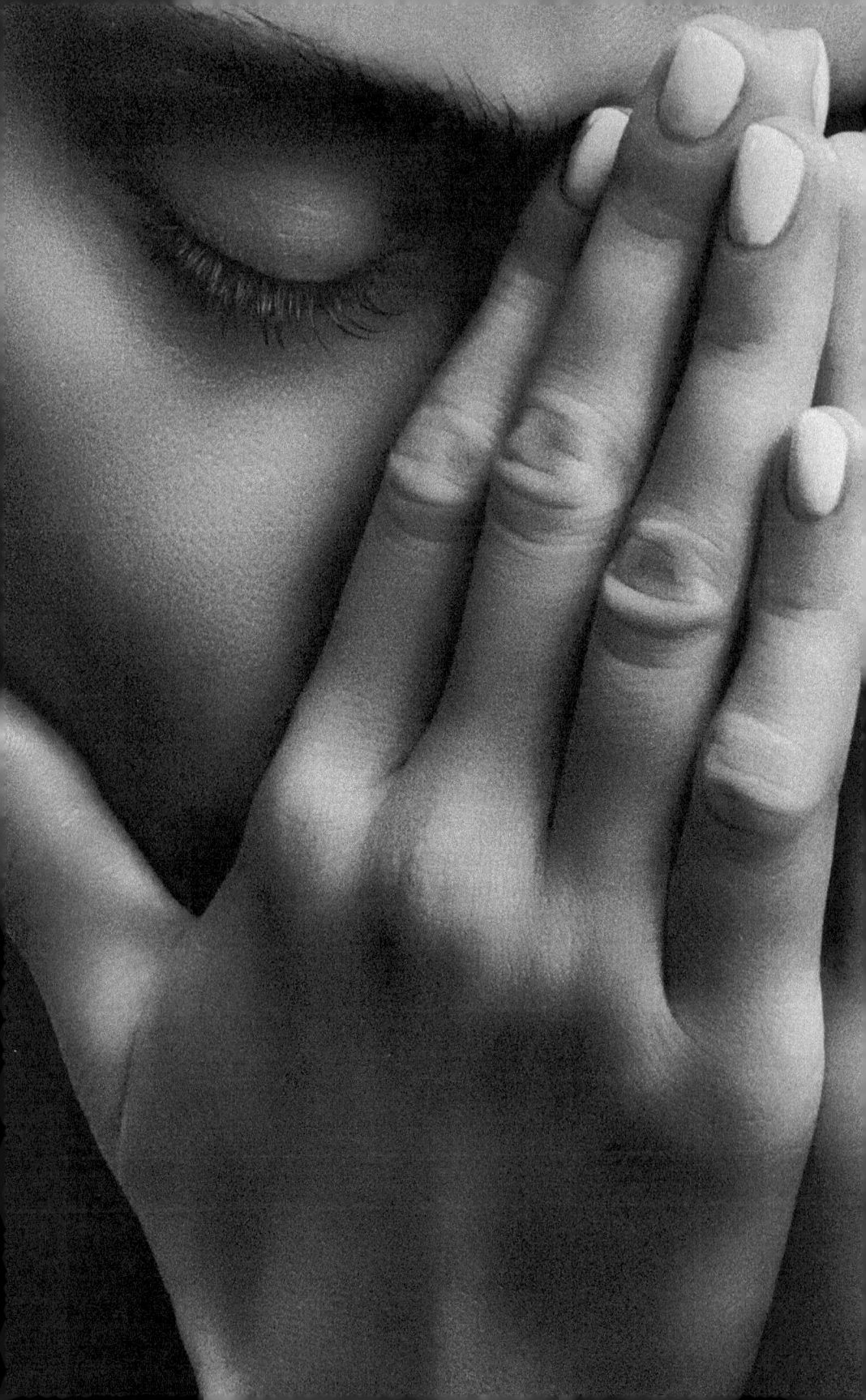

CHAPTER FIVE
Is Your Depression a Symptom of PTSD?

Depression and PTSD are two peas in a pod. Most people who suffer PTSD describe some degree of depression and vice versa.

In this chapter, I will reveal the hidden causes of depression that are not widely known by doctors and mental health care professionals.

According to Healthine.com, the most common forms of depression are Major Depressive Disorder, Persistent Depressive Disorder, Bipolar Disorder*, Seasonal Depression (SAD), Postpartum Depression and Psychotic Depression.

The most common symptoms of depression are extreme irritability over seemingly minor things, anxiety and restlessness, trouble with anger management, loss of interest in activities, including sex, fixation on the past or on things that have gone wrong, and thoughts of death or suicide.

Depression is also accompanied by physical symptoms, such as insomnia or oversleeping, debilitating fatigue, increased or decreased appetite, weight gain (weight gain in depressed people is conventionally assumed to be caused by overeating, when, in fact, there is research proving that many depressed people gain weight not from overeating but due to the elevated cortisol levels that are associated with depression) or loss, difficulty concentrating or making decisions, and unexplained aches and pains.

Regarding the causes of depression, mainstream medicine cites:

- Brain chemistry imbalances
- Hormone imbalance
- Genetic predisposition
- Low self-esteem
- Anxiety disorder
- Borderline personality disorder

PTSD (remove this)

- Physical or sexual abuse
- Chronic diseases like diabetes, multiple sclerosis and cancer
- Abuse of alcohol or drugs
- Certain prescription medications
- Family history of depression
- Age, gender, race and geography

Treatment

According to the World Health Organization, less than 50 percent of those suffering depression receive treatment. This is an especially disturbing statistic considering that untreated depression often leads to other conditions that severely impact a person's life, including alcohol or drug use, headaches and other chronic aches and pains, phobias, panic disorders and anxiety attacks, poor school or work performance, disturbed family and intimate partner relationships, social isolation, excess weight, weight loss, increased risk of heart disease and type 2 diabetes, self-mutilation and attempted suicide or suicide.

The most common treatments are antidepressant medications and psychological counseling. Psychotherapy has a lower rate of relapse than medications (26. 5 percent versus 56.6 percent).

According to the American Psychiatric Association, a combination of antidepressants and psychological counseling is more effective.

Other therapies include: repetitive transcranial magnetic stimulation and light therapy (especially for Seasonal Depression) and electroconvulsive therapy (ECT) which is used to treat intractable depression that hasn't responded to medications.

Little Known Causes of Depression

From the start of my professional career 37 years ago, I bucked the Western practice of masking mental health and physical ailments with medications.

In the early 80s, my first professional position was at a private inpatient psychiatric hospital. There I began researching the underlying causes of every mental and physical health condition, including depression.

I was appalled to see how many patients kept returning to the hospital year after year. Clearly the medications and therapy were missing the mark for most people.

For example, I'll never forget one of my first patients, a man named Chester. For decades, four times a year, he was hospitalized and administered ECT for his intractable depression. Clearly, even the ECT wasn't doing it.

I sensed that something he was consuming on a daily basis was disturbing his brain chemistry. I already knew that allergies could impact any organ in the body. I began to wonder if allergies could trigger brain chemistry imbalances and mood disturbances such as depression. Something told me that Chester's brain was negatively reacting to wheat. So, I asked Chester to run an experiment and eliminate wheat. Low and behold his depression cleared in a week, and he never returned to the hospital again!

Another patient, a 250-pound veteran, was depressed and suffering a porn addiction. He admitted to masturbating multiple times a day. It was clear to me that he was masturbating in an attempt to raise his endorphin levels, which temporarily shifted his brain chemistry and lifted his depression for a brief time. In our sessions, I uncovered buried anger toward his mother. When he was a child, his mother told him that if he was angry with her, she would drop dead of a heart attack. Her emotional blackmail resulted in his "sitting" on his anger. Buried anger often morphs into depression for several reasons. The anger has to go somewhere, and if it can't go outward toward the object of the anger, it gets misdirected and turned back on the self. Depression can be a form of mental self-attack. Also, the energy needed to push down or suppress anger literally depresses the psyche.

I'll never forget the day that I helped this man to unearth his anger toward his mother. He began to shake and looked like a volcano about to erupt. Suddenly, this huge ex-soldier began to weep like a baby. The next thing I knew, he landed in my lap, crying profusely as the rage poured out of him. Low and behold, his depression lifted!

Another patient was depressed and suffering panic attacks. I questioned her to determine whether her attacks occurred at a particular time of day. Sure enough, they occurred at the same time each day, which led me to suspect she had hypoglycemia (low blood sugar). As I came to realize, mood often follows blood sugar fluctuations. When the blood sugar drops too low, an anxiety or panic attack can occur; or the mood can drop, triggering a greater sense of depression. This observation led me to suspect that the reason why many depressed people feel most depressed in the morning is due to blood sugar levels being lowest upon awakening.

I even suspect that the high and low mood fluctuations of Bipolar Disorder may be linked to blood sugar fluctuations.

Another man I treated suffered panic attacks, but only on airplanes—and he didn't have a fear of flying. When I heard this, I suspected and confirmed chemical sensitivities were the culprit.

Yet another man I treated suffered a life-long depression that was worse in the winter and growing progressively worse as he aged. Lower serotonin levels in winter due to less natural light and low vitamin D levels were obviously part of the cause of his depression. But when I learned that his problem had worsened with age, I was sure that diminished testosterone levels were aggravating his underlying seasonal depression. I also suspected that low thyroid was a factor in his depression—which lab tests revealed. How many millions of people suffer undetected or subclinical hypothy-roidism as an unrecognized cause of their depression?

What about intestinal flora imbalances/dysbiosis, and the rampant leaky gut/intestinal permeability** that nearly every person suffers as a result of consuming pesticide-tainted wheat and corn, genetically modified grains, overheated cooking oils, sugar, high-fructose corn syrup and packaged foods, all of which damage the gut lining.

Research now proves that neurotransmitters and hormones are integrally linked to mood-regulation.[30]

We also know that gut microbes produce serotonin, the feel-good neurotransmitter. And, astonishingly, 90 percent of our serotonin production happens in the gut![31]

Surely, the world-wide epidemic of gut dysbiosis and leaky gut is a major factor in the ever-rising depression epidemic. In fact, there is research showing that low magnesium alters the gut microbiota and causes depression.[32]

The bottom line (pun intended) is this: Dysbiosis and a damaged gut lining are a direct cause of depression. This means if you are depressed, the first line of defense is to improve your diet and correct your microbiome.

Last but not least, perhaps the least known hidden cause of depression is low magnesium.

It stands to reason that depression has reached epidemic proportions because magnesium deficiency has also reached epidemic proportions.

There is a great deal of scientific research proving that low magnesium levels cause depression and that magnesium supplementation quickly reverses depression. In fact,

one published NIH research article entitled "Rapid recovery from major depression using magnesium treatment" found that major depression was eliminated in less than 7 days using 125-300 mg of magnesium glycinate and taurate.[33]

As I've said previously, oral magnesium results in 30 percent absorption at best. And, many people can't tolerate oral magnesium at all. So, rather than treating depression with oral magnesium, it makes sense to use transdermal magnesium, which bypasses the gut entirely and insures absorption.

Oral magnesium causes diarrhea and gastrointestinal symptoms at worst, and 30% absorption at best.[34]

Transdermal magnesium provides superior cellular absorption.[35, 36, 37, 38, 39]

If you or someone you love is suffering depression, in addition to exploring all the hidden factors I mentioned in this chapter, I encourage you to make transdermal magnesium your first line of depression therapy.

Beware of stopping antidepressant drugs cold turkey, which can cause rebound depression and anxiety, as well as other health risks. And, be sure to wean yourself off medication under a doctor's supervision.

I close this chapter by reassuring you that your depression is curable. Please don't give up hope. Just keep exploring all the variables I mentioned until you uncover the puzzle piece(s) that fits for you.

*Bipolar Disorder is commonly treated with lithium. Lithium competes with magnesium or, more accurately, lithium is the body's plan B when there is not enough magnesium available because both magnesium and lithium can occupy GABA receptor sites to create calmness.[40, 41]

** Our beneficial gut bacteria produce their own fatty acids, which are then incorporated into the endothelial lining of the gut, helping to protect and maintain the gut lining. The more we lose the fatty protection, the leakier our membranes become. Fat is protective, but in sequestering the toxins it can become overloaded and breakdown (oxidize) which then leads to inflammation. This is why detox and anti-oxidant support, in conjunction with magnesium, are so important in preventing decay and decomposition.

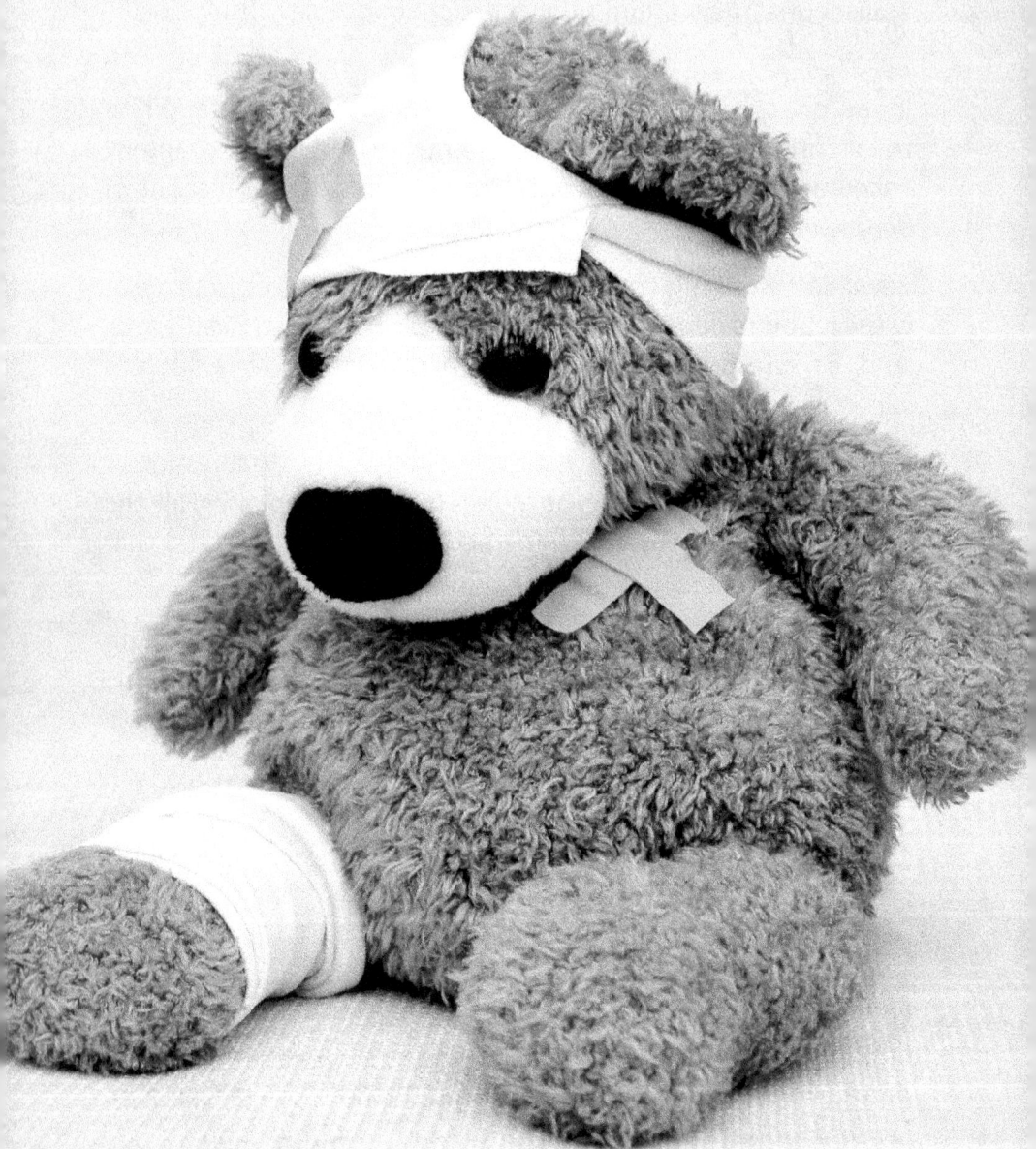

CHAPTER SIX
Physical Pain and PTSD

Does your body hurt most or all of the time?

Do you suffer from throbbing, burning, stinging or stabbing pain?

Do you have headaches?

Or chronic neck or back pain?

Do your bones hurt?

Are your muscles stiff and sore?

Does pain make it hard or impossible to perform daily activities like dressing or bending?

Is exercising impossible or are you laid up with pain after you physically exert?

Do you regularly take OTC or prescription pain medicines or anti-inflammatory drugs?

Are you using drugs or alcohol to numb your pain?

Are you taking OTC or prescription pain meds on a daily basis?

Are you taking more than the prescribed dose of OTC or prescribed medicines?

Do you feel guilty or useless as a result of your pain?

Have you lost your sex drive?

Is pain wrecking your sleep?

Are you unable to work or on disability because of your pain?

Is pain making you irritable and causing relationship difficulties?

And, last but not least, does the pain make you feel like you don't want to live?

If you said yes to any of the above questions, you're not alone.

According to the CDC: "1 in 5 adults suffer chronic pain. 8% had high–impact chronic pain defined as limiting life or work activities on most days or every day during the past 6 months, according to a CDC report. Chronic pain is a growing public health concern in the United States, costing an estimated $560 billion each year for medical care, lost productivity, or disability services, according to a 2011 Institute of Medicine (IOM) report. In addition to interfering with day-to-day activities, chronic pain is associated with dependence on opioids, anxiety and depression, and a poor quality of life, according to the CDC report. Previous estimates of chronic pain among US adults varied between 11% and 40%. With the goal of fulfilling a recommendation of the National Institutes of Health's National Pain Strategy, the CDC analyzed data from the 2016 National Health Interview Survey to get a more precise estimate of chronic pain prevalence."[42]

Approximately one in three Americans suffer some form of chronic pain in their lifetimes, and about one quarter of them are not able to do day-to-day activities because of their chronic pain.

And this next statistic is staggering: Between 80% and 90% of Americans experience chronic problems in the neck or lower back.[43]

What exactly is Chronic Pain Syndrome?

According to Columbia University, "Unlike acute pain, this condition doesn't go away after your initial injury or illness has healed. It's marked by pain that lasts longer than six months and is often accompanied by anger and depression, anxiety, loss of sexual desire, and disability."[44]

Pain comes in many forms.

There is acute pain following an accident, illness or surgery.

And there is chronic pain stemming from bone, muscle or nerves (neuropathic) and caused by either vascular (vessels) issues, inflammation, obstruction or distension.

Chronic pain can also be caused from consumption of GMOs and gluten.

The following is a list of common and little known conditions that cause Chronic Pain Syndrome, including drug side-effects (statins can cause a condition called statin myalgia) drugs for osteoporosis and Paget's disease, fluoroquinolones (a class of antibiotics), retinoids (for skin conditions, like Accutane for acne), Trintellix (an antidepressant), repetitive stress injury, IBS, IBD, Crohn's disease, ulcerative colitis, MS prodrome, AIDS, Complex Regional Pain syndrome (CRPS), Interstitial Cystitis (IC), mitochondrial disease, traumatic brain injury, trigeminal neuralgia, cancer, lymphoma, stroke, shin splints, bone spurs, osteoarthritis, Rheumatoid arthritis (RA), autoimmune diseases, lupus or SLE, Ehlers-Danlos syndrome and the hypermobility spectrum disorders, ligament stress syndrome associated with antibiotic use and adrenal fatigue, claudication (from impaired blood flow), Facioscapulohumeral Muscular Dystrophy, gallbladder disease, gout, acute pancreatitis, endometriosis, acid reflux, kidney stones, diabetic neuropathy, unexplained neuropathy and neuroinflammation, ulcers, endometriosis, post-surgical pain, post-traumatic pain following an injury or accident, nerve damage, migraine and cluster headaches, shingles, frozen shoulder, heart attack, Sickle cell disease, broken bones, sciatica, slipped disc, myelopathy (spinal cord impingement), syphilis, Lyme disease, chronic immune activation after infection, trigger point pain, fibromyalgia, and a rare condition called Scleroderma*.

When you conduct an Internet search under: Chronic Pain Syndrome, the following comes up: "Treatment can help, but this condition can't be cured."

So how exactly does Western medicine treat Chronic Pain Syndrome?

Here is what Columbia University, one of the world's most respected "top"/remove this word academic and research medical establishments says on their website regarding how to treat Chronic Pain Syndrome:

"These are possible treatment options:

- Behavior modification, such as cognitive behavioral therapy
- Acupuncture
- Psychotherapy
- Biofeedback
- Hypnosis
- Occupational therapy
- Physical therapy
- Relaxation techniques, such as meditation, visual imagery, or deep breathing

- Medications to help control pain, such as anti-inflammatory drugs, antidepressants, anticonvulsants, and opioids
- Nerve blocks
- Surgery to treat any underlying conditions"[45]

I must take a moment to discuss the travesty that pervades the Western medical establishment's widespread use of anti-depressants in treating chronic pain.

And, yes, this practice is widespread:

"At doses lower than those needed to treat depression, antidepressants can relieve chronic pain in conditions ranging from diabetic neuropathy, migraine and tension headaches, to osteoarthritis and fibromyalgia. In fact, they are so effective, that antidepressants are the mainstay for treating chronic pain."[46]

Need I reiterate? Anti-depressants are the medical mainstay for treating chronic pain.

Why?

Because there is a pervasive belief in the medical community that, "Among severe chronic pain patients, 94% had depression. This and much other research demonstrate that severe and disabling chronic pain is a symptom associated with serious psychosocial distress, often a major mental disorder such as clinical depression."[47]

Let's break this down.

Mainstream medicine believes that depression is the underlying cause of physical pain (isn't pain, itself, depressing?).

Added to this belief is the fact that women, who statistically suffer more pain, have been told for centuries, and continue to be told, that their pain is due to stress, anxiety or depression, otherwise known as "it's all in your head" or psychosomatic.[48]

Let's take a moment to talk about the psychosomatic label.

How does the medical establishment treat a depressed or anxious person, especially a woman, who also suffers chronic pain?

Sooner or later, that person ends up in a psychiatrist or other mental health professional's office. Mental health practitioners diagnose patients using the *The Diagnostic and Statistical Manual of Mental Disorders, 5th Edition* (DSM-5). It's important to note that the DSM-5 only mentions the term "chronic pain" a few times. On page 813 of the DSM-5, it states: "Some individuals with chronic pain would be appropriately diagnosed as having Somatic Symptom Disorder, with predominant pain."[49]

The Mayo Clinic's website describes symptoms of Somatic Symptom Disorder as:

- Specific sensations, such as pain or shortness of breath, or more general symptoms, such as fatigue or weakness
- Unrelated to any medical cause that can be identified, or related to a medical condition such as cancer or heart disease, but more significant than what's usually expected

The key phrase is "unrelated to any medical cause that can be identified."

Just because your doctor doesn't know what's causing your pain doesn't mean it's psychosomatic, or all in your head!

The Mayo Clinic website goes on to say:

"Pain is the most common symptom, but whatever your symptoms, you have excessive thoughts, feelings or behaviors related to those symptoms, which cause significant problems, make it difficult to function and sometimes can be disabling."[50]

Apart from the disabling nature of pain itself, why wouldn't someone suffer excessive thoughts, disabling feelings and be excessively worried about pain that his/her doctor cannot figure out!

The medical mainstream's belief that anxiety or depression is the cause of pain is ridiculous and dangerous because this thinking leads to first-line treatment of pain using anti-depressant and anti-anxiety drugs.

Here's the key point: Which comes first—pain, leading to anxiety and depression, or depression and anxiety leading to pain? In the end it doesn't matter, because the key point is that all these conditions are due to low Mg.

Why?

Because there is one underlying factor that can cause depression and anxiety and chronic pain:

Low magnesium!

In short, there is ample research proving that low magnesium causes chronic pain and that magnesium reverses all kinds of pain from all different origins:[51]

Intravenous magnesium may relieve or reverse chronic complex regional pain syndrome type 1 (CRPS-1).[52]

The role of magnesium in alleviating pain is clear.[53, 54, 55, 56]

Yet, despite the research, the mainstay of Chronic Pain Syndrome treatment is anti-depressants and other drugs.

What a dangerous abomination!

Especially considering that we know that prescription drugs lower magnesium levels.[57]

Let me break this last point down: The drugs prescribed for pain (which itself is caused by low magnesium), lower magnesium levels further, worsening the underlying cause of the pain condition. This is just plain nuts.

I have to wonder if the reason anti-depressants stop working as time passes is precisely because the drugs themselves lower magnesium, which worsens depression and pain. Worsening depression due to lower magnesium leads to an increased dosing of the anti-depressant drug, which lowers magnesium levels even more, and creates a vicious cycle of ever-increasing depression and pain.

Why do we not see magnesium even mentioned by prominent medical establishment's websites as the first-line of treatment for pain syndromes?

For one thing, most doctors don't take a single course in nutrition, meaning they're not trained to think of nutrients instead of medicine.

The mainstream medical mindset is to prescribe drugs to treat symptoms.

As I said previously, the stress associated with the Coronavirus (COVID-19) has left millions of people depleted of magnesium, and pushed the world population into what I call a *Global PTSD Pandemic Stress Syndrome*.

It's important to note here that approximately 15% to 35% of patients with chronic pain also have PTSD.[58]

Because we know that stress depletes magnesium and triggers PTSD, and we know that low magnesium also triggers Chronic Pain Syndrome, it stands to reason that our entire PTSD-plagued world is currently or will likely soon be suffering Chronic Pain Syndrome.

As a final note, it's important that you not fall prey to the erroneous mainstream method of testing magnesium levels. Healthline.com says:

"The symptoms of magnesium deficiency are usually subtle unless your levels become severely low. Deficiency may cause fatigue, muscle cramps, mental problems, irregular heartbeat and osteoporosis. If you believe you may have a magnesium deficiency, your suspicions can be confirmed with a simple blood test."[59]

Wrong!

Once again, most doctors do not know that research proves that serum (blood) tests are not an accurate measure of magnesium levels.[60]

This is because the body needs to maintain a very specific level of magnesium (in a very narrow range) in the bloodstream in order for the heart to continue beating! To keep blood levels high enough, the body pulls magnesium from the organs and cells, causing undetected cellular low magnesium. Hence why a hair analysis, which is a long-term blueprint of body chemistry, is a better way to test magnesium levels. But hair analysis is only a general guide. Symptomology is a better indicator of deficiency.

Where does serum magnesium testing leave the millions who suffer chronic pain? Your doctor sends you home saying you have excellent magnesium levels, when you're actually suffering rampant cellular magnesium deficiency causing all kinds of health problems and symptoms, including pain. By the way, by the time a blood test reveals low magnesium, you're practically on death's door, literally one beat away from a heart attack!**

As a final note, it's important to not get caught up in diagnostic labels because PTSD, anxiety, depression and Chronic Pain Syndrome all share the same underlying factor: low magnesium.

I want to leave you with hope. Last year I treated the 87-year-old mother of a patient of mine. This woman is an MD who had been bed-ridden for four years due to spinal pain. We sprayed the **Elektra Magnesium** spritz oil on her back. Within a couple hours, she was up and out of bed for the first time in four years!

If you or someone you love is suffering Chronic Pain Syndrome, PTSD, depression and/or anxiety, do not despair. There is a proven way to manage and reverse these conditions by correcting your magnesium deficiency using transdermal magnesium, which is the most bio-available and absorbable form.

* Almost all pain syndromes and conditions are directly or indirectly linked to low magnesium.

** In addition to hair analysis, which is a non-invasive way to test long-term magnesium levels and ratios, the Exatest (http://exatest.com/Research.htm) is an oral cheek swab, which provides an accurate current measure of intracellular magnesium levels. If you're working with an alternative or open-minded doctor, you can request that he/she order this test for you.

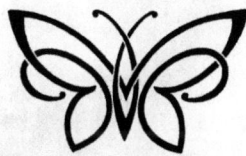

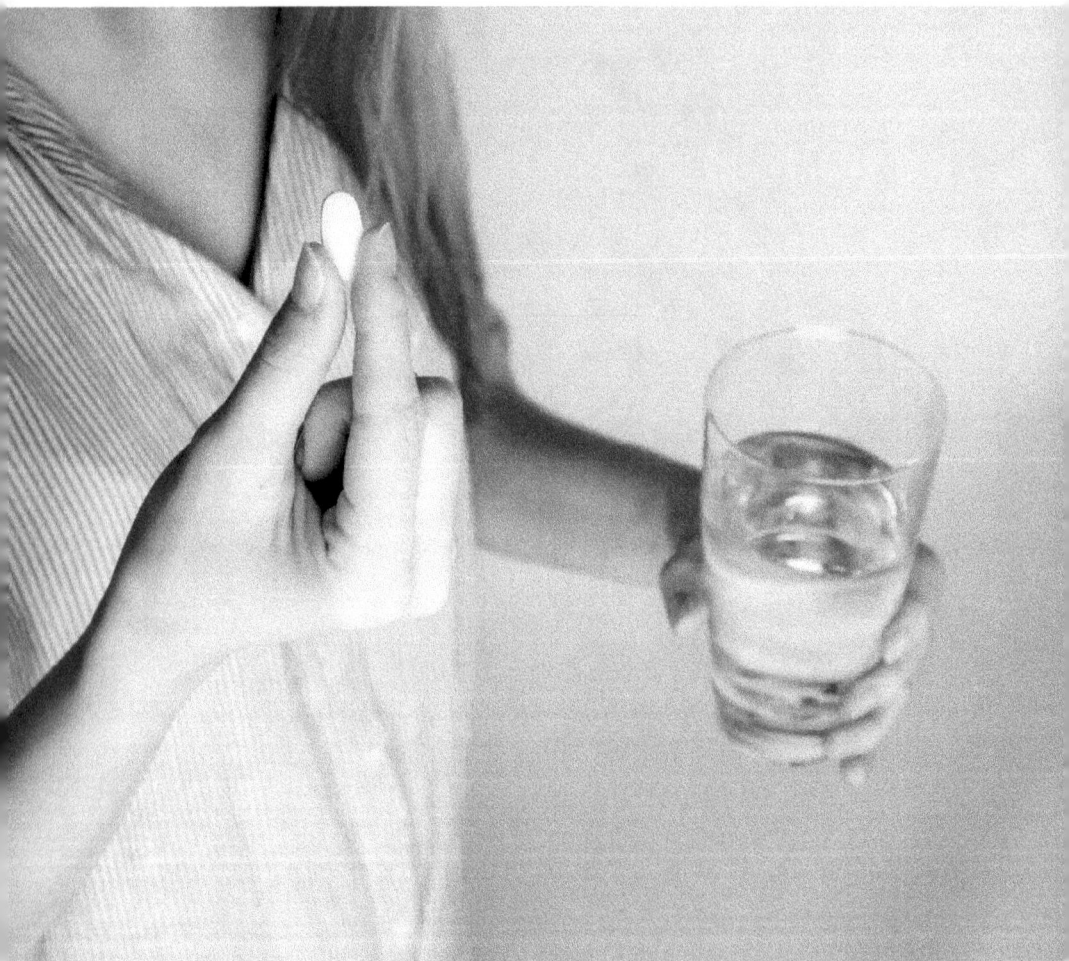

CHAPTER SEVEN
Could Your Addiction be PTSD in Disguise?

Do you use prescription, over-the-counter or street drugs on a daily basis?

Do you find yourself powerless to control your use of these drugs?

If you said yes to my above questions, you are not alone.

"Drug use is on the rise in this country and 23.5 million Americans are addicted to alcohol and drugs. That's approximately one in every 10 Americans over the age of 12 – roughly equal to the entire population of Texas. But only 11 percent of those with an addiction receive treatment. It is staggering and unacceptable that so many Americans are living with an untreated chronic disease and cannot access treatment," said Dr. Kima Joy Taylor, director of the Closing the Addiction Treatment Gap (CATG) Initiative.

According to the National Survey on Drug Use and Health (NSDUH), 19.7 million American adults (aged 12 and older) battled a substance use disorder in 2017.[61]

Almost 74% of adults suffering from a substance use disorder in 2017 struggled with an alcohol use disorder.

About 38% of adults in 2017 battled an illicit drug use disorder.

That same year, one out of every eight adults struggled with both alcohol and drug use disorders simultaneously.[62]

In 2017, 8.5 million American adults suffered from both a mental health disorder and a substance use disorder, or co-occurring disorders.

Drug abuse and addiction cost American society more than $740 billion annually in lost workplace productivity, healthcare expenses, and crime-related costs.

Genetics, including the impact of one's environment on gene expression, account for about 40% to 60% of a person's risk of addiction.

Environmental factors that may increase a person's risk of addiction include a chaotic home environment and abuse, parent's drug use and attitude toward drugs, peer influences, community attitudes toward drugs, and poor academic achievement.

Teenagers and people with mental health disorders are more at risk for drug use and addiction than other populations.[63]

In 1956, the American Medical Association (AMA) declared alcoholism an illness, and in 1987, the AMA and other medical organizations officially termed addiction a disease.

The term addiction does not only refer to dependence on substances such as heroin or cocaine. A person who cannot stop taking a particular drug or chemical has a substance dependence.

Some addictions also involve an inability to stop partaking in activities, such as gambling, eating, or working. In these circumstances, a person has a behavioral addiction.

Addiction is a chronic disease that can also result from taking medications. The overuse of prescribed opioid painkillers, for example, causes 115 deaths every day in the United States.

When people are addicted, they cannot control how they use a substance or partake in an activity, and they become dependent on it to cope with daily life.

Every year, addiction to alcohol, tobacco, illicit drugs, and prescription opioids costs the U.S. economy upward of $740 billion in treatment costs, lost work, and the effects of crime.

Most people start using a drug or first engage in an activity voluntarily. However, addiction can take over and reduce self-control.[64]

The Following Are the Most Common Types of Addictions:

- Alcohol
- Coffee
- Drugs (over-the-counter, prescription, illegal)
- Food
- Gambling
- Internet/Social Media/Cell Phone
- Love*
- Rage*
- Sex/Pornography
- Shopping
- Tobacco/Nicotine
- Video games
- Work

Let's take a moment to discuss two of the less known addictions listed above: love and rage addictions.

Love chemicals can become addictive. According to research, attraction reduces the hormone serotonin, which is involved in appetite and mood. It's interesting to note that obsessive-compulsive disorder is linked to low serotonin levels which may explain why those newly in love can become overwhelmed with feelings of obsession for the love object.

You or someone you know may be addicted to rage, if the following signs are present:

- Verbal, Physical, Or Emotional Abuse Towards Others
- Excessive Cursing
- Name Calling
- Threatening Behavior
- Pointing and Yelling
- Sarcasm, Even When It Is Uncalled For
- Throwing Objects at Others
- Experiencing Temper Tantrums
- Bragging About Power and Control
- Criticizing and Degrading Others with Blunt, Aggressive Comments
- Road Rage
- Mixing Anger with Substance Abuse
- Unpredictable Behavior
- Denying Anger Outbursts
- Fantasies of Revenge

In the same way that substances trigger brain chemical rushes, so too does the expression and expulsion of anger. Like any addiction, anger can induce discharge of dopamine, epinephrine and norepinephrine—also referred to as adrenaline and noradrenaline.[65]

The Following are the Physical Signs of Addiction:

- Lack of concern over physical appearance/personal hygiene

- Disrupted sleep patterns, including insomnia
- Over-active or under-active (depending on the drug)
- Repetitive speech patterns
- Dilated pupils, red eyes
- Excessive sniffing and runny nose (not attributable to a cold)
- Looking pale or undernourished
- Clothes do not fit the same
- Weight loss
- Change in eating habits
- Unusual odors or body odor due to lack of personal hygiene[66]

The Following are the Behavioral and Social Signs of Addiction:

- Secretive or dishonest behavior
- Poor performance and/or attendance at work or school
- Withdrawing from responsibility and socializing
- Losing interest in activities, hobbies or events that were once important to you
- Continuing to use the substance, or engage in certain behaviors, despite the negative consequences that these cause
- Trying but failing to reduce or stop misusing a substance, or engaging in certain behaviors
- Missing work/school
- Work/school problems
- Missing important engagements
- Isolating/secretive about activities
- Disrupted sleep patterns
- Legal problems
- Relationship/marital problems
- Financial problems (e.g. always needing money)
- Conversations dominated by using or drug/alcohol related topics

The Following are the Psychological and Emotional Signs of Addiction:

- Mood swings
- Irritability/Argumentative
- Increased temper
- Tiredness
- Paranoia
- Defensiveness
- Agitation
- Inability to focus or concentrate
- Poor judgment
- Memory problems
- Diminished self-esteem and self-worth
- Feelings of hopelessness
- Exacerbation of any existing mental health conditions such as depression, anxiety or stress
- Inability to deal with stress
- Loss of interest in activities/people that used to be part of their lives
- Obnoxious behavior
- Silly behavior
- Confused easily
- Denial
- Rationalizing—Offering alibis, excuses, justifications, or other explanations for their using behavior
- Minimization—Admitting superficially to the problem but not admitting to the seriousness or full scope of the behavior or consequences
- Blaming—Placing the blame for the behavior on someone else or some event
- Diversion—Changing the subject to avoid discussing the topic

The Following are the Three Cs of Addiction:

- Loss of control over the amount and frequency of use
- Craving and compulsive using
- Continued use in the face of adverse consequences[67]

The Western Treatment for Addictions

Now let's look at how the Western medical establishment treats addictions.

The first line of treatment in substance addiction treatment is detoxification, which consists of clearing a substance from the body and limiting withdrawal reactions.

In 80 percent of cases, a treatment clinic will use medications to reduce withdrawal symptoms, according to the Substance Abuse and Mental Health Services Administration (SAMHSA).

If a person is addicted to more than one substance, that person is often prescribed different medications to reduce withdrawal symptoms for each of the substances to which he/she is addicted.

Using pharmaceutical drugs to "cure" other drug addictions is just plain crazy. For example, Methadone is the drug that is most often used to treat heroine and opioid addictions. Meanwhile, Methadone is, itself, addictive. In other words, the Western drug addiction treatment protocols consist of trading one addition for another.

Why? Methadone is big-business for Big Pharma.

Interestingly, when you search the medical literature, there is a dearth of research discussing just how addictive Methadone is. Yet, there are many detox clinics that treat the widespread epidemic of Methadone addiction caused by our Western treatment protocols.[68]

In addition to the use of drugs to treat addiction, the following are additional mainstream treatment protocols:

- Cognitive-behavioral therapy (CBT), which helps people recognize and change ways of thinking that are associated with drug abuse behaviors
- Multi-dimensional family therapy, designed to help improve family function around an adolescent or teen with a substance-related disorder
- Motivational interviewing, which maximizes an individual's willingness to change and make adjustments to behaviors
- Motivational incentives that encourage abstinence through positive reinforcement[69]

Other common recommendations include:

- Individual psychotherapy to teach the client how to handle the triggers that lead to substance abuse
- Group counseling sessions with other clients who also suffer from PTSD and an addictive disorder
- Couples therapy or family counseling to strengthen relationships and educate family members about the disorder
- Membership in a 12-step group to strengthen the client's support network
- Medication therapy with anti-addiction drugs or psychotherapeutic medications (antidepressants or anti-anxiety medications)

As an aside, I have always been skeptical of the efficacy of cognitive-behavior therapy (CBT) in treating addictions because addictive behaviors are caused by underlying chemical imbalances. When the brain is under the influence of these chemical imbalances, it is impossible to trick or train the brain to think or act differently. Until the underlying chemical imbalance is fixed, the thoughts and the behaviors that spring from these chemical imbalances are nearly impossible to alter. I'm reminded of an alcohol-addicted patient who I treated decades ago. Alcohol craving and addiction is a symptom of low GABA levels in the brain, which triggers anxiety and addictions. In addition to craving alcohol when GABA is low, those with low GABA also tend to crave and become addicted to nicotine and sugary, fatty foods, all of which raise GABA. This explains why alcohol addicts often become addicted to sugar when they give up drinking. The only way I could resolve my patient's panic attacks and addictive behaviors was to prescribe GABA. My point is prescribing Methadone for drug addiction is treating a symptom not the cause of the addiction, which is the underlying brain chemical imbalance.

"When studying brain chemical imbalances associated with addiction, we must discuss dopamine, the hormone that's linked to the brain's reward pathway—and that means controlling both the good and the bad. We experience surges of dopamine for our virtues and our vices. In fact, the dopamine pathway is particularly well studied when it comes to addiction. The same regions that light up when we're feeling attraction light up when drug addicts take cocaine and when we binge-eat sweets. For example, cocaine maintains what is called 'dopamine signaling' for much longer than usual, leading to a temporary 'high'. In a way, attraction is much like an addiction to another human being. Similarly, the same brain regions light up when we become addicted to material goods as when we become emotionally dependent on our partners. And addicts going into withdrawal are not unlike love-struck people craving the company of someone they cannot see."[70]

Addiction and the Microbiome

We know that disturbed neurotransmitters are the underlying cause of all addictions. Yet, Western medicine ignores the fact that the microbiome is where 95% of our neurotransmitter chemicals are made. In other words, our gut is the seat of the neurotransmitter imbalances that lead to addiction.

Because of our modern Western diet and lifestyle, we're dealing with a universal microbiome disruption, which leads to leaky gut/intestinal permeability. Then, we prescribe drugs to mask these imbalances, drugs that further disrupt the microbiome, creating more brain chemical imbalances and addiction! (Note: magnesium is also essential to healing and sealing the gut wall.)

"Dopamine is one of the brain's neurotransmitters affected by virtually all drugs of abuse; however, there are many other chemical messengers that can be impacted as well. Some drugs may increase the presence of a particular brain chemical by stimulating its production, while others may block them from being reabsorbed. Neurotransmitters are typically either excitatory or inhibitory, meaning that they either provide stimulation or nervous system depression, respectively."[71]

How Neurotransmitters Affect
Health and Happiness

"Dopamine is a neurotransmitter that plays a key role in mood, motivation and drive, desire, satiety and pleasure. This has earned dopamine the distinction of being labeled the feel-good chemical, but other neurotransmitters can also have a pleasure/reward effect. Endorphins are considered 'pleasure chemicals' because a boost in endorphin levels contributes to making us feel better when we exercise, have sex or fall in love, and reduces our perception of pain. Serotonin plays a role in relaxation, sleep and appetite. Gamma-aminobutyric acid, or GABA, has a calming effect and, thus, also relaxes us. Norepinephrine is another neurotransmitter that is released when we fall in love, and also plays a role in concentration, alertness and energy, particularly related to how we respond to stressful situations. Acetylcholine's role is to help us remember things and process information. Glutamate has many different roles, but is particularly important in regulating brain function—its neurotransmitter system supports cognition, learning and memory."[72]

How Addiction and Dopamine Neurotransmitters are Related

"The mechanism by which our brain's reward center regulates neurotransmitters undergoes a change when we drink alcohol or take certain drugs, and this is how these chemicals can play a role in addiction. In most people, there is a temporary shift in neurotransmitter levels after we have a drink or other substance, but those levels soon shift back to normal after we metabolize it. In other people, the brain's response to a change or super-charged surge of neurotransmitters brought on by alcohol or other drugs catalyzes a response from the brain's reward center that says, 'I have to have some more of that!' This same response can occur with addictive behaviors like gambling, where a person feels a rush of excitement with the anticipation of winning (even when they don't win)."[73]

"For people who have a predisposition for addiction, the circuitry in the brain's reward center changes. Addiction and dopamine neurotransmitters result in a 'reward' to certain substances or stimuli. Over time and with repeated exposure, the person begins to crave more of the substance or activity that produces the positive feelings or relief from negative feelings. But the brain is just one part of the story. Addiction has many contributing factors—from genetics (addiction can run in families) to socio-economic status, one's environment and any pre-existing mental health disorders. (For example, we know there is a high prevalence of depression, trauma and other problems among drug users.) All of these elements play a role in how we respond to alterations in neurotransmitters levels."[74]

The following is a summary of how different substances affect us:

"Let us assume that the stage is set for addiction. The addiction and the dopamine neurotransmitters, as well as other factors, motivate a person to take, continue taking, and become dependent upon a drink or drug. Here's how different substances affect the brain and its neurotransmitters:

- Alcohol is thought to affect several neurotransmitter systems, including those for GABA, glutamate, serotonin, dopamine and endorphins, resulting in either a sedative or an excitatory effect, depending on extent of use.
- Benzodiazepines (Valium, Xanax, Ativan, Rivotril) impact GABA, resulting in a sedative effect."
- Opioids (painkillers like Vicodin, Percocet, OxyContin, morphine and the street version of heroin) impact endorphins and other naturally occurring opioids in our system, modulating our reactions to pain and altering functions like mood control, hunger and thirst.
- Amphetamines (Adderall, Ritalin, Dexedrine) are often used to combat fatigue, impact dopamine and some glutamate receptors, resulting in increased energy and feelings of excitability.
- Cocaine boosts dopamine levels, producing cravings and dependency on the drug.

- It also affects serotonin, leading to feelings of confidence, and norepinephrine, increasing energy.
- Ecstasy/Molly (MDMA) is a psychostimulant that simultaneously works as a stimulant and a hallucinogen. It affects norepinephrine, dopamine and serotonin, leading to a combined effect of increased energy, euphoria and lowered inhibitions in relating to other people.
- Marijuana (cannabis) affects both dopamine and the neurotransmitter anandamide, which is involved in regulating mood, memory, appetite, pain, cognition and emotions. (fix missing space here) The resulting sensations include mild euphoria, relaxation and amplified auditory and visual perceptions."[75]

I would like to add that benzos occupy the GABA receptors so that the body produces less and less of its own GABA. When GABA is low, the body craves sugary and fatty foods, nicotine and alcohol, all of which raise GABA levels. The problem with alcohol and sugar (after the short-term calming effect) is that their metabolism produces excessive acids— free radicals—and that over-stimulates the glutamate release, causing jitters and explosive energy down the line because there is not enough natural GABA (or magnesium that can help to produce more GABA. Magnesium is the Rolls Royce choice to feed the body what is needed.) The metabolism of sugars also consumes huge amounts of magnesium and lowers magnesium stores, which cause the release of more stress hormones, and the cycle continues to worsen.

Eventually all this leads the body to crash into depression because the metabolism is shot. When the brain doesn't receive enough energy, it craves stimulants like nicotine, caffeine or alcohol to fire-up. Does the addiction get worse as the person chases more dopamine hits in the form of caffeine drinks, adrenaline rushes from gambling, risky sex, etc., all of which provide a temporary "lights-on" energy burst for the brain because the metabolism is failing? But these highs precede a crash to extreme lows, and the body keeps losing equilibrium. Too much sugar and stimulants have to go somewhere—have to be dealt with by the liver, eventually leading to more overload and toxicity, acidity, inflammation, pain and eventually cell death if there is not enough magnesium and antioxidant counterbalance.

PTSD and Addiction

According to dualdiagnosis.org, 52 percent of males and 28 percent of females with PTSD meet the lifetime criteria for alcohol abuse or dependence, according to findings on post-traumatic stress disorder in the National Comorbidity Survey, published in 1995 in the Archives of General Psychiatry (Kessler et al.). When it comes to drug abuse, statistics from the same study show that 35 percent of men and 27 percent of women with PTSD meet the criteria.

Endorphin withdrawal plays a part in the use of alcohol or drugs to control PTSD. When an individual experiences a traumatic event, his or her brain produces endorphins—neurotransmitters that reduce pain and create a sense of well-being—as a way of coping with the stress of the moment. When the event is over, the body experiences an endorphin withdrawal, which has some of the same symptoms as withdrawal from drugs or alcohol:

- Anxiety
- Depression
- Emotional distress
- Physical pain
- Increased cravings for alcohol or drugs

According to Alcohol Research & Health, many of those with PTSD will turn to alcohol as a means of replacing the feelings brought on by the brain's naturally produced endorphins. But the positive effects of alcohol are only temporary.

With increased use of alcohol, the individual can become chemically dependent on the drug. He or she will need more alcohol or drugs to produce those numbing effects. Eventually, dependence can turn into addiction, which is characterized by compulsive use of the substance, tolerance to the drug and an insistence on abusing the drug in spite of its devastating effects.

The use of alcohol to numb PTSD symptoms leads to a vicious cycle. Drinking alcohol worsens the fear and anxiety of PTSD, which leads to a release of endorphins.

Where does magnesium figure in all this?

Once again, research shows that low magnesium is directly linked to addictions and, not surprisingly, also linked to reduction in addiction and dependency:

For example, one NIH published research says,

"Addiction is a dysregulation of brain reward systems that progressively increases, resulting in compulsive drug use and loss of control over drug-taking. Addiction is a brain disease. There is evidence that magnesium deficit is involved in addiction to various addictive substances (heroin, morphine, cocaine, nicotine, alcohol, caffeine, and others). Magnesium is involved in all the stages of addiction.

Magnesium deficit enhances the vulnerability to psycho-active substance addiction. Stress and trauma reduce the brain magnesium level and at the same time favor addiction development. In experimental studies, administration of magnesium while inducing morphine dependence in rats reduced the dependence intensity.

Magnesium reduces the NMDA receptor activity and the glutamatergic activity. Because stress and trauma induce hypomagnesemia with increased vulnerability to addiction, magnesium intake by people who are under prolonged stress could be a way to reduce this vulnerability and the development of addiction to different psychoactive substances. Anxiety and depression appear to be associated with increases in drug-related harm and addictive substance use. Magnesium anxiolytic effect could be important for the anti-addictive action. Addiction is characterized by relapses. Magnesium deficiency may be a contributing factor to these relapses."[76] Insert line break here

Another study focused exclusively on PTSD and addictions:

"Addiction to different substances is considered to be a psychiatric disorder. Magnesium reduces the intensity of addiction to opiates and psychostimulants (cocaine, amphetamine, nicotine, and others). It also decreases the auto-administration of cocaine and the relapse into cocaine and amphetamine intake, as well as reducing the experimental addiction to morphine, cocaine and other substances in animals. In heroin addicts, alcohol consumers and other drug abusers, the plasma and intracellular magnesium concentration is lower compared to healthy subjects. We consider that one of the mechanisms by which magnesium reduces the consumption of some highly addictive substances is its moderate effect of stimulating the reward system.

However, other main mechanisms involved in magnesium's action are the reduction of dopamine and glutamate release at presynaptic terminals in the brain, the decrease of NO synthase activity, the stimulation of GABAergic system activity, the reduction of postsynaptic NMDA receptor activity, and the reduction of some neuromediators released by Ca^{2+} and acting at calcium channels. Apart from the action of magnesium ions during emerging addiction, administration of this cation after the appearance of withdrawal syndrome reduces the intensity of the clinical symptoms. There are data that show that stress increases the vulnerability of people to develop addiction to different substances, and also reduces drug-free time and increases the incidence of relapse in heroin addicts. Stress increases catechol-amine release and stimulates magnesium release from the body. This decrease in magnesium concentration is one of the important factors that hastens relapse."[77]

The research is clear. Addictive behaviors, substance abuse and PTSD are linked to neurotransmitter imbalances, which are themselves linked to low magnesium. The research also shows that magnesium reverses these addictions and PTSD.

It's an abomination that Western addiction treatment protocols do not incorporate this essential mineral in the treatment protocols. Instead, Western addiction treatment consists of prescribing drugs to suppress addictive behaviors, drugs that further lower magnesium and worsen the underlying cause of addiction.

I close this chapter by issuing a call to arms: Rather than use drugs to treat symptoms of addiction, substance abuse and PTSD, it's time to use magnesium to treat and reverse the underlying neurotransmitter imbalances that cause addictions and PTSD.

Note: Cannabis can occupy our endocannabinoid receptors of the gut-brain connection and vagus nerve, and mimic our natural endocannabinoids.[78]

CHAPTER EIGHT
Could PTSD Be Causing Your Sagging Sex Life?

Recently, I began reflecting on a hunch that most people with PTSD also suffer sexual dysfunction.

This idea came to me because I know that PTSD is caused by HPA-Axis dysfunction. (The HPA-Axis refers to the primary neuro-biochemical stress response network that involves both the central nervous and endocrine systems. HPA-Axis dysfunction, hippocampal volume, and endogenous opioid function are technical terms that describe total adrenal burnout. Burnout is the end result of the body being trapped too long in fight-flight mode—also known as sympathetic arousal.)

Because I know that HPA-Axis dysfunction is linked to sexual dysfunction, I was sure that I would find a lot of research discussing the concurrence of PTSD and sexual dysfunction.

But, when I began digging into the research, I was alarmed by what I uncovered: a notable lack of scientific research on the topic of PTSD and sexual dysfunction.

I found one small mention of the concurrence of PTSD and sexual dysfunction on the VA website:

"PTSD impairs sexual functioning across multiple domains: desire, arousal, orgasm, activity, and satisfaction. The most commonly reported problems were erectile dysfunction, premature ejaculation, and overall sexual disinterest."[79]

Though it is more common than not for those with PTSD to experience sexual dysfunction in all aspects of sexual functioning including desire, arousal, activity, orgasm and satisfaction, I began to wonder why the American Psychiatric Association (APA) and the DSM-5 don't even mention sexual dysfunction in their extensive list of PTSD diagnostic criteria symptoms, especially considering that research shows that 85% of male combat veterans diagnosed with PTSD reported erectile dysfunction, compared with a 22% rate among male combat Veterans without any mental health diagnosis.[80]

Another study of 90 male combat veterans with PTSD found more than 80% were experiencing sexual dysfunction.[81]

To complicate matters, most of the limited research focuses on sexual dysfunction among male veterans.

What about female veterans and sexual dysfunction?

According to the VA, "Combat is not the only trauma experienced in the military. Nearly 24 percent of female Veterans seeking VA health care report a history of military sexual trauma, or MST. In the review study, this group of women displayed negative sexual consequences above and beyond the effects of civilian sexual assault. Though the researchers say the reason for the differing rates is not yet fully understood, one explanation could be that unlike in civilian situations, survivors of MST often are required to continue working with their attacker. Researchers say this could compound the stress and make them more vulnerable to developing sexual dysfunction. Moreover, Veterans with PTSD, whether as a result of combat, MST, or both, may also be more likely to misuse alcohol and other illicit substances. This further increases the risk of sexual dysfunction."[82]

PTSD and Sexual Dysfunction in Non-Military Populations

According to statistics, the lifetime prevalence of PTSD for women who have been sexually assaulted is 50% (10). Moreover, sexual assault is the most frequent cause of PTSD in women, with one study reporting that 94% of women experienced PTSD symptoms during the first two weeks after an assault.[83, 84]

"Research findings also indicate that sexual dysfunctionality is often misdiagnosed and not immediately taken care of. Conclusion: The severity of the pathology regarding sexual dysfunctionality calls for immediate planning and coping."[85]

Another researcher said, "Difficulties in sexual desire and function often occur in persons with post-traumatic stress disorder (PTSD), but many questions remain regarding the mechanisms underlying the occurrence of sexual problems in PTSD."

This same researcher postulated that sexual dysfunction in PTSD is related to an "inability to regulate and redirect the physiological arousal needed for healthy sexual function away from aversive hyperarousal and intrusive memories." Remove extra character space that was here[86]

To restate the above in lay terms, the author is stating that those with PTSD get stuck in hyperarousal (which is another way to say HPA-Axis Dysfunction) and this physiological overdrive blocks healthy physiological arousal mechanisms.

Link Between HPA-Axis and the Sympathetic Nervous System

According to Harvard University, "The HPA axis relies on a series of hormonal signals to keep the sympathetic nervous system— the 'gas pedal'—pressed down. If the brain continues to perceive something as dangerous, the hypothalamus releases corticotropin-releasing hormone (CRH), which travels to the pituitary gland, triggering the release of adrenocorticotropic hormone (ACTH). This hormone travels to the adrenal glands, prompting them to release cortisol. The body thus stays revved up and on high alert. When the threat passes, cortisol levels fall. The parasympathetic nervous system—the 'brake'—then dampens the stress response."[87]

It is important to note that under normal circumstances, when the stressful event is over, the gas pedal is lifted, the body shifts from sympathetic arousal to parasympathetic arousal, and cortisol levels drop back into normal range.

But, the return to "normal" physiology doesn't happen in the case of PTSD.

Think of PTSD as stress that never ends because PTSD creates ongoing emotional and physical reactions such as:

1. Recurrent, involuntary, and intrusive distressing memories of the traumatic event(s).
2. Recurrent distressing dreams in which the content and/or affect of the dream are related to the traumatic event(s).
3. Dissociative reactions (e.g., flashbacks) in which the individual feels or acts as if the traumatic event(s) were recurring. (Such reactions may occur on a continuum, with the most extreme expression being a complete loss of awareness of present surroundings.)
4. Intense or prolonged psychological distress at exposure to internal or external cues that symbolize or resemble an aspect of the traumatic event(s).

5. Marked physiological reactions to internal or external cues that symbolize or resemble an aspect of the traumatic event(s).[88]

Sadly, the intrusive memories, dreams and flashbacks, the same emotional and physical reactions that characterize PTSD, paradoxically keep reactivating the chemical imbalances that caused PTSD in the first place. This reactivation process keeps the chemical imbalance of PTSD alive indefinitely.

How HPA-Axis Dysfunction Turns off Sexuality

To complicate matters, long-term stress creates hormonal shifts that put the brakes on sex drive and performance.

It stands to reason that when we get locked in overdrive, or sympathetic arousal, we are not in the mood to get down!

The shutdown of our sexual drive in the face of HPA-Axis/ sympathetic arousal is adaptive, dating back to prehistoric times when we needed to react with lightning speed—to flee or fight dangerous prey.

When prehistoric man was on high-alert, fighting for survival, fists—and drawers—needed to stay up. It hardly made sense for prehistoric man to be thinking about dropping trou when a tiger was baring down on him! He needed to be thinking: How do I stand a better chance of not ending up in the bottom of the beast's belly; should I flee or fight? As you can see, the automatic reaction to turn-off the sex drive in the face of stress is a built-in survival adaptation.

Once the tiger trotted off, the caveman's physiology returned to normal, insert comma allowing his body to switch from sympathetic arousal back to parasympathetic mode, which is also known as rest, digest and—get down—mode!

But in the case of PTSD, the accelerator pedal stays in overdrive for a long period of time. As a result, the body becomes a cortisol production factory.

How Excess Cortisol Screws Up Sexuality

When I searched the scientific literature, I found a lot of research on how men and women respond differently to stress, and what types of stressors trigger HPA-Axis dysfunction in men and in women.

But I didn't find a lot of scientific research on how HPA-Axis dysfunction affects male versus female sexuality.

What exactly happens to male and female sexuality when stress doesn't go away?

We know that cortisol is the main hormone of the HPA-Axis and the primary stress hormone.[89]

"The stress response is controlled by the hypothalamic-pituitary-adrenal (HPA) axis. The hypothalamus directs the pituitary, or 'master gland,' which is found as a small protrusion off of the hypothalamus. The pituitary controls the secretion of hormones throughout the body. Depending on the messages it receives from the hypothalamus, it may signal the adrenals to secrete cortisol, a stress hormone, or the gonads to secrete sex hormones. Stress hormones can impact and interfere with sexual function at all three levels of the HPG axis: at the brain, pituitary, and gonads."[90]

We also know that cortisol reduces the production of the male sex hormone testosterone. For most people with long-lasting stress or PTSD symptoms, testosterone production is reduced.

According to Norwegian doctor, psychiatrist, and clinical sexologist Haakon Aars, "Testosterone is the sex hormone with the greatest significance to sex drive in both men and women. This means that your sex drive decreases due to completely logical physiological reasons."[91]

How Stress and PTSD Affects Female Sexuality

A recent study of women complaining of low or absent sexual desire found their low desire may be linked to hypothalamic-pituitary-adrenal (HPA) axis dysregulation.

There is a prevailing belief that low testosterone is linked to low sex drive in both men and women. One research showed that it is low DHEA that is linked to sexual dysfunction in women.

"In contrast to the extensive research investigating, but not finding an association of women's sexual desire with their testosterone levels, many studies have found lower serum levels of DHEA in women reporting low or absent sexual desire."[92]

"However, in addition to stress hormones, the adrenals can also produce DHEA, a sex hormone. DHEA is a precursor to both testosterone and estrogen. Although testosterone is often thought of as a male hormone, women also have it in smaller amounts, and it has a strong impact on libido.

In menstruating women, the ovaries are the major source of testosterone, but the adrenals contribute via their production of DHEA. After menopause, the adrenals become critical to a woman's supply. If a woman has adrenal fatigue, not only will her production of stress hormones decrease, but her testosterone—and her libido—will too.

Higher stress is associated with reduced sexual functioning in general. Women who had higher levels of cortisol (the stress hormone) and lower levels of DHEA (the sex hormone) after watching an erotic movie experienced less physiological arousal than women with a lower cortisol/DHEA ratio. Prolonged stress has been shown to decrease sexual response in women, and women with greater levels of chronic daily stress report more sexual complaints.

Stress can interfere with sex on a psychological level, too. Cognitive distraction (thinking or worrying about problems) interferes with sexual functioning. So, if you are ruminating about multiple stressors, it will be difficult to put your full attention on either your partner or your own sensations and responses."[93]

Eliminate "this drive/"

Link between Stress, HPA-Axis Dysfunction and Sexual Dysfunction in Men

When it comes to arousal in men, there is a delicate dance going on between the sympathetic and parasympathetic nervous systems. If a man is too stressed out, as is the case with PTSD, he is locked in sympathetic arousal mode, which triggers excess cortisol. As I said, cortisol has disastrous effects on male sexuality.

Sexual Desire

Chronic stress, ongoing stress over an extended period of time, can affect testosterone production, resulting in a decline in sex drive or libido, and can even cause erectile dysfunction or impotence.[94]

Reproduction

Chronic stress can also negatively impact sperm production and maturation, causing difficulties in couples who are trying to conceive. Researchers have found that men who experienced two or more stressful life events in the past year had a lower percentage of sperm motility (ability to swim) and a lower percentage of sperm of normal morphology (size and shape), compared with men who did not experience any stressful life events.[95]

In summary, the chronic stress associated with PTSD causes excess cortisol production. Excess cortisol lowers the production of testosterone and DHEA, both of which are linked to suboptimal sexual performance in men and women, respectively.

How to Reverse Sexual Dysfunction that Accompanies PTSD

Whenever treating a condition, it's vital to treat the cause rather than the symptom. So, rather than throwing aphrodisiac herbs at your testicles or ovaries, let's truly get to the bottom of the problem—if you'll pardon my pun.

Sexual dysfunction associated with PTSD is linked to HPA-Axis dysfunction, which triggers excess cortisol production, which, in turn, lowers the hormones needed for sexual arousal and function.

We know that magnesium supplementation reverses HPA-Axis dysfunction and PTSD.

Research also shows that magnesium directly reduces cortisol levels. Because excess cortisol is the underlying cause of the sexual dysfunction that the majority of PTSD sufferers face, it stands to reason that magnesium should be the first line of treatment for those with PTSD who also suffer sexual dysfunction.

If you are suffering sexual dysfunction and PTSD, don't despair. Magnesium is a natural, drug-free remedy for both conditions.

Note: In some people, oral magnesium can cause diarrhea and gastrointestinal symptoms at worst, and 30% absorption at best; so, when treating sexual dysfunction and PTSD, I recommend using *Elektra Magnesium*, which bypasses digestion and instantly enters your bloodstream.

CHAPTER NINE
Is Your Derailed Digestion Due to PTSD?

Are your guts in a knot?

Do you suffer from gas, bloating, constipation, diarrhea, reflux, acid indigestion, GERD, IBS, IBD, colitis, Crohn's disease, Celiac disease, ulcers or SIBO?

Did you know that all these digestive ills are triggered by chronic stress and PTSD?

In this chapter, I will attempt to untangle the very complex web of interconnections between stress and the digestive system.

To simplify, when we are stressed, the body switches to sympathetic arousal mode, also known as the fight-flight response. In my first Hay House book, *Kiss Your Fights Goodbye*, I discussed how this response is triggered in the face of relationship conflict and fighting. In *Kiss Your Fights Goodbye*, I outlined how to recognize if one's relationship fighting has triggered this chemical imbalance by identifying the various visible physical manifestations of sympathetic arousal/fight-flight mode.

What I didn't discuss in *Kiss Your Fights Goodbye* was all the other invisible, yet very dangerous physical consequences of not only relationship distress, but stress of any kind.

As I have said previously, stress causes a massive depletion of magnesium. Magnesium loss is associated with HPA-Axis dysfunction, which is the scientific term for the inability to disengage from the sympathetic arousal/fight-flight mode so you can fully relax. Studies have shown that as magnesium levels drop, the release of adrenalin and cortisol increases, and vice versa. Magnesium therefore has a dampening effect on stress hormones.

When this mineral deficiency becomes chronic and pervasive, the digestive system malfunctions and becomes sluggish. Short term flight-flight response is well tolerated, as long as we have an optimal supply of nutrients, particularly magnesium. This shutdown was adaptive and very useful during prehistoric times when the caveman was faced with dangerous prey. In extreme life-threatening situations, the caveman's blood was shunted away from the stomach and into the muscles, so that he could flee or fight the predator.

As adrenalin and cortisol stress hormones got pumped into the system, those hormones moved calcium into the heart, leg and arm muscles, and also provided more blood for oxygen supply, to enable strong muscle contraction and very quick movements—as in run fast! Then, after the danger passed, his body shifted back into parasympathetic mode, also called the rest and digest mode. In this state, magnesium moved back in and calcium moved out so that the muscles could relax again, and more blood returned to his stomach muscles so that he and his family could chow down on the tiger he skewered, produce the required stomach acid, and fully digest the meal with no issue.

In modern times, stress is so pervasive that we end up in a constant state of fight-flight, meaning our digestion is perpetually running on low reserves and minimum capacity— just like when your computer runs on safe mode to conserve energy and resources. Imagine what the constant revving of your car engine would do. Of course, it needs a chance to cool down, rest and recover to keep working properly too.

To summarize how the nervous system directly impacts digestion: The parasympathetic nervous symptom (PNS) is designed to produce the rest and digest, among other responses in your body, including the calm that allows your body to repair itself.

The PNS stimulates digestion through increasing the blood flow directly to your digestive tract. As opposed to the sympathetic nervous system (SNS) response, your salivary gland is stimulated, increasing the saliva that contains enzymes that begin the initial chemical process of digestion.

Another function of the PNS is to increase peristalsis, which is the constriction and relaxation of the intestine (sphincter) muscle. This motion pushes the contents through the intestines. As such, peristalsis is essential to food and nutrient absorption. Without it, natural waste elimination is not possible.[96]

Impairment of digestion is synonymous with sluggish motility, that is, slow transit of food through the digestive pipework.

What happens when our food travels through our digestive system too slowly?

As the perpetual pumping out of stress hormones wears down the adrenals (part of the HPA-Axis), it also affects the metabolic performance of the thyroid in that system, as they work in tandem. We need the thyroid to be working properly in order to produce the right amount of stomach acid (hydrochloric acid and pepsin enzymes). The thyroid must have enough iodine, magnesium and selenium for proper function. To make stomach acid and digestive enzymes you also need additional nutrients including chloride, B group vitamins, zinc, and vitamin K. These are resources that get depleted during stress.

Less stomach acid means food takes longer to digest and tends to hang around longer in the stomach, causing fermentation and production of gases and bloating, eventually erupting as esophageal reflux (GERD). Low stomach acid can become a negative feedback loop as the impairment to digestion means you are getting shortchanged on the nutrients you need to support the thyroid and make stronger stomach acid and enzymes.

Once the food chyme is mulched enough it passes through from the stomach to the small intestine, but can at this stage still contain too many bad bacteria that should have been killed by the stomach acid. This is the main way people develop SIBO – Small Intestinal Bacterial Overgrowth. These bacteria tend to proliferate in the small intestine, which should generally be a low-bacterial environment. They chow down on your food and rob you of some of that nutrition, often competing for your iron supply. This can cause symptoms of anemia and low energy, which is another way to slow down the digestive tract and transit of food.

The longer food takes to transit through the intestines, the more it dries up as feces, as these microbes start to produce the methane that is associated with constipation. Around we go on the merry-go-round, getting robbed of nutrients, breeding bad bacteria that upset the microbiome and make more acids and free radicals that can eat away at the intestinal lining causing the leaky gut symptoms of Irritable Bowel Syndrome (IBS). This condition eventually ends up triggering other down-stream diseases, with the whole chain of events and symptoms being a result, initially, of exhaustive and unrelenting stress.

The situation can get worse, with food that sits too long in the gut and begins to putrefy and rot. This leads to overgrowths (bacterial, fungal, and/or parasitic) because these bugs thrive in the acidic environment of putrefied food. When overgrowths throw the gut microbiome out of whack, ulcers, IBS, IBD, ulcers, colitis, and Crohn's can develop due to the increasing level of acids and the low oxygen environment.

The bad bugs (anaerobic low-oxygen-loving) thus crowd out the good bugs/healthy digestive flora (aerobic, oxygen-loving). In a healthy gut environment, the aerobic alkaline bacteria maintain the integrity of the gut mucosal lining and also release enzymes that trigger normal peristalsis when it's time to take out the garbage—that is, when it's time to poop the refuse.

One of the important functions of good flora (predominantly Bifidobacterium and Lactobacillus species and their friends), is digestive motility. In other words, good bacteria help maintain the normal muscular activity of the small bowel, which creates waves that move the food contents of the intestine through the gut. So, as you can see, with low stomach acid and worsening motility the bad microbes take over and cause more trouble.

The pathogenic bugs can feed on and chew up our protective mucin lining, producing more acidic wastes and eventually causing sensitivity and burning pain as the lining becomes more raw and exposed (as in ulcerative colitis). At this stage, if you eat complex carbohydrates, like vegetables or porridge that bring in fiber for motility and help create mucin, these prebiotics can also fuel the activity of the pathogenic bugs, thereby setting off a major vicious cycle.

As an aside: large meals and high fat diets slow transit time. The latest research shows that the popular high fat/keto diet slows transit and encourages dysbiosis. Good carbs (complex carbohydrates) feed the garden, bring in vitamins, minerals, fiber and water to support the gut lining mucin layer, thereby fertilizing the good bugs, which can then choke out the bad guys. Without the right carbs, the bad gut bugs win the war, acidify the intestinal environment, and age us faster. They can become dominant monocultures. The best diet is one that offers a variety of foods with a good balance of fats, protein and complex carbohydrates (including fermented foods). The variety of foods brings a variety of nutrients and a variety of beneficial gut bacterial species. The more variety, the better.

The keto diet may for a period of time keep the bad bacteria quiet, but it is too extreme because of its deficiency of plant fibers and accompanying minerals and hydration. A diet deprived of fibers (or dietary MACs) is associated with an increased incidence of colitis and pathogenic infections, while a regular consumption of dietary fibers (laboratory diet containing ~15% of dietary fibers from minimally processed grains and plants) had a preventive effect, suggesting in this way that fiber plays a crucial role in contributing to the presence of a protective mucus barrier.[97]

Depletion of the mucin layer is associated with metabolic syndrome, diabetes or obesity. These are down-stream effects of chronic acidity and difficulty to detox or to buffer the acids with enough antioxidants. The bacterial metabolic waste acids erode collagen proteins and the mucosal layer of the gut lining. As more of the mucin layer is lost, leaky gut/intestinal permeability is the inevitable outcome.

When we reach this stage, nutrient absorption is compromised, toxins gain entry to the body's interior where they shouldn't be, and that sets off a cascade of disease.

With gut permeability in full swing, we begin to absorb undigested food particles (also due to low stomach acid), which triggers abnormal immune reactions such as allergies and excess histamine production. At this stage of the game, we may also develop worsening chronic fatigue, fibromyalgia, and other hypothyroid conditions.

Chronic infections (another stressor) also fatigue the adrenals. I have come to believe that the catch-all diagnoses of adrenal fatigue/chronic Lyme are actually undetected gut infections.

Because over 80% of your immune system resides in your gut, "the health of your gut bacteria and the health of your immune system are vitally linked. When your gut bacteria is balanced, your immune system is also balanced. But when it's out of balance, so is your immune system."[98]

Given what's going on in the world, most people are in constant inflammatory overdrive, living in a state of hyper-sensitivity, hyper-inflammation and hyper-vigilance as the body struggles to rebalance the pH from the acid invasion of the bad bugs. But the enemy has too many weapons of acidity. Because our immune systems are on overdrive, we fall into more metabolic stress, which causes more cortisol production, more fight-flight response, and ever worsening digestive ills. There has to be a way to find the reset button.

Another side effect of gut dysbiosis is, as the gut lining loses protection from the mucin layer, we can develop interstitial cystitis (IC). This is when the bugs migrate into the interstitial region between the bladder and bowel. It can also happen if the kidney is compromised and struggling to eliminate waste products.

We mustn't forget that the good bugs make important neurotransmitters like serotonin, GABA and B12, which keep us calm and happy. As I've said before, mood disturbances, such as depression and anxiety, are linked to bowel imbalances. This is how connected the Gut-Brain Axis is. It brings us around again to the effects of stress and magnesium depletion, because our beneficial bacteria are also dependent on magnesium for metabolism.

A balanced gut microbiome is also the home of our hormone production, which has powerful effects on growth, energy, ability to handle stress, sex drive, etc. The gut is also the home of most of the immune system—essentially your white blood cells that defend us against invaders.

Migrating Motor Complex (MMC) dysfunction is a disruption to normal peristalsis and digestive motility, which is linked to Vagus Nerve dysfunction. It is now established that a disturbed microbiome with dominant pathogens can inhibit normal bowel motility.

"Some may secrete messenger molecules that travel through the blood to the brain. Other bacteria may stimulate the vagus nerve, which runs from the base of the brain to the organs in the abdomen. Bacterial molecules might relay signals to the vagus through recently discovered "neuropod" cells that sit in the lining of the gut, sensing its biochemical milieu, including microbial compounds. Each cell has a long "foot" that extends outward to form a synapselike connection with nearby nerve cells, including those of the vagus." 99 See article on the psychobiome, an exciting new frontier in research.

Bad bugs can also cause ileocecal valve dysfunction as the gas pressure from the bad bugs forces the valve open, allowing bad bacteria to migrate backwards to the small intestine, making SIBO symptoms worse. It's like the whole intestinal system loses its rhythm of smooth muscle movement control. The excessive gas produced by the bad bugs can back up all the way to the lower esophageal sphincter (LES) and force this valve open as well, causing acid indigestion, reflux and GERD.

What's more, bug infections can damage the villi of the small intestine, which project into the intestinal cavity, greatly increasing the surface area for food absorption and adding digestive secretions. The villi number about 10 to 40 per square millimeter (6,000 to 25,000 per square inch) of tissue. Recently, it's been demonstrated that healthy villi are needed for proper motility. So, again, by damaging the villi, bugs find yet another way to disrupt motility, creating another mechanism for their continued survival.

I have to take a moment to also mention how glyphosate figures into the equation. Glyphosate is known to kill off beneficial bacteria, while favoring the pathogens, which then wreak havoc on the gut lining. This impairs mineral absorption, causing the nervous system and immune system to become super sensitive, fragile, and easily triggered.

It's like being primed and pumped up, ready for the stress response so that the slightest hair trigger can set us off. Glyphosate chokes cells by inhibiting oxygen metabolism and magnesium, and so affects every cell in the body. When oxygen is in short supply the body panics and adrenalin and cortisol release goes up. These stress chemicals produce more acids, which further depletes oxygen.

In other words, glyphosate is a chemical stress causing PTSD by robbing the body of nutrient access, which affects the gut microbiome and a whole cascade of downstream side effects, including neurotransmitter production, immune system and endocrine function. Energy metabolism becomes sluggish and the body's natural detox mechanisms weaken. It's a disastrous revolving door—a poisonous trap. Going organic makes a lot of sense when you understand the dangers and consequences of these types of chemicals in our food supply.

Antibiotics, chlorinated fluoridated drinking water, pharmaceutical drugs, and the highly processed, sugar-laden Western diet also feed the acid environment and therefore encourage proliferation of more bad bugs. We become a bit like a walking compost heap, acidifying and breaking down.

I have to mention here that the pervasive prescribing of acid-lowering drugs, such as proton pump inhibitors (PPIs), worsens the problem. We need stomach acid to kill bad bugs. By lowering stomach acid, we create an even more fertile environment for pathogens to thrive, especially helicobacter pylori.

I like Joe Dispenza's war analogy to describe the battle going on inside our bodies.

"For a moment, think about the dispersion of an army. If the majority of an army at war is dispersed to, say, a western front, this leaves the eastern front vulnerable because the once-balanced strategy of defense has been diminished. The same goes for your body's inner environment.

If you're tapping all of your body's resources for some emergency in your outer world, it makes sense then that there's no energy in your inner world to not only make white blood cells—which are your body's internal army designed to fight infection and other diseases—but to allow them to function properly.

Over time, because the body is in an emergency state, the immune system, digestive system, and the cardiovascular system dial down because the energy required to maintain its optimal effectiveness is being dispersed to other parts of the body. In other words, the body is essentially conserving energy, which causes the immune cells to have less of a response. This redistribution of energy also alters a person's blood flow from the brain and the heart.

As blood flow constricts, energy leaves the heart and the brain to attend to the adrenal center. Now the person is on high alert all the time, and that person is more in their animal nature than in their divine nature."[100]

In summary, our inner and outer worlds in modern times of high-density industrialized conditions are under a siege of never-ending sympathetic arousal/fight-flight response/HPA-Axis dysfunction.

This stress siege creates an acidic environment that attracts mucin-devouring bugs to move into the gut and literally eat us for lunch, thus eroding the protecting gut lining, which develops into leaky gut syndrome.

When under siege, we don't have enough energy left to tap into our hearts and spiritual natures, because the immune system is constantly triggered to keep fighting off the pathogenic invaders. This hyperstimulation can also lead to autoimmune disorders, which further drain our batteries.

I reiterate what I have said elsewhere in this book: Stress depletes magnesium levels; magnesium loss triggers HPA-Axis dysfunction; HPA-Axis dysfunction causes PTSD, and can even be seen as synonymous with it (as in the **Global PTSD Pandemic Stress Syndrome**). Research has consistently shown that supplementing with magnesium reverses PTSD, helping the body to return to balance in the parasympathetic mode.

Magnesium is the master key mineral electrolyte that controls stress hormones and calcium. It is the sparkplug of the electro-magnetic energetic circuit that releases constriction and opens our hearts to raise our energetic field in fuller communion with Spirit. It's all about energy and life force, and when stress and parasites are stealing our energy we're always chasing our tail, but never getting ahead of the game. So, it becomes hard to function in balance physically, emotionally and spiritually—and therefore to live a joyous and fulfilling life.

There is a worldwide epidemic of digestive woes caused by stresses of all kinds (including chemical stresses), which leads to nutritional deficiencies due to compromised digestion. The world is suffering PTSD (and the **Global PTSD Pandemic Stress Syndrome**), which is synonymous with magnesium deficiency.

How can we unplug from this horrible treadmill? I recommend that you seek out a professional to guide you in reviewing your diet in relation to gut health, so that you are promoting a healthy gut microbiome. To counteract growing acidity, you need a lot of antioxidant support. But changes to the microbiome can take a long time. Our foods have also become quite depleted in magnesium, which supports antioxidant activity.

While you are getting your gut microbiome back in order using diet, you can also do some other things to manage stress better, such as meditation, deep breathing exercises, listening to calming music, watching comedy, regular moderate aerobic exercise, hugging your pets and loved ones, and getting out into nature more. These destressing activities will slow down the loss of magnesium and conserve your supplies.

Another way to calm the body is by drinking mineral water. Water is life, and we are made mostly of water. We are like a big walking fish tank, and that tank needs to be cleaned regularly with fresh clean water. You need good hydration because water delivers Hydrogen2 and Oxygen for cell metabolism, buffering acids, and all the flowing rivers in the body that transport nutrients in or take wastes out: All require a good supply of water.

Drinking water fortified with magnesium delivers a better electrical charge due to water structuring, and this makes water more hydrating for cells. If you are feeling low in energy, depressed or anxious for no apparent reason, it could very well be a signal that your body is just dehydrated and missing magnesium and water supply.

However, for those who are very magnesium-depleted, there is an extra way to get ahead faster. You can absorb magnesium ions transdermally using dissolved magnesium chloride salts in bathing and foot soaking, which help the body to detox via skin. Magnesium sulfate (Epsom salt) also delivers magnesium, but much less than magnesium chloride, and the sulfates can irritate and dry out skin—especially the sensitive skin types. Magnesium chloride, however, is skin hydrating and softening.

You can also apply Magnesium Cream, Oil or Lotion as skin care products and for muscle relaxation massage. This will help to relax the body quickly. Remember that relentless stress is the enemy, the all-consuming fire, but magnesium can extinguish it so the body can relax and chill out. It is very liberating to know this happens perfectly naturally and without drugs or chemical interventions.

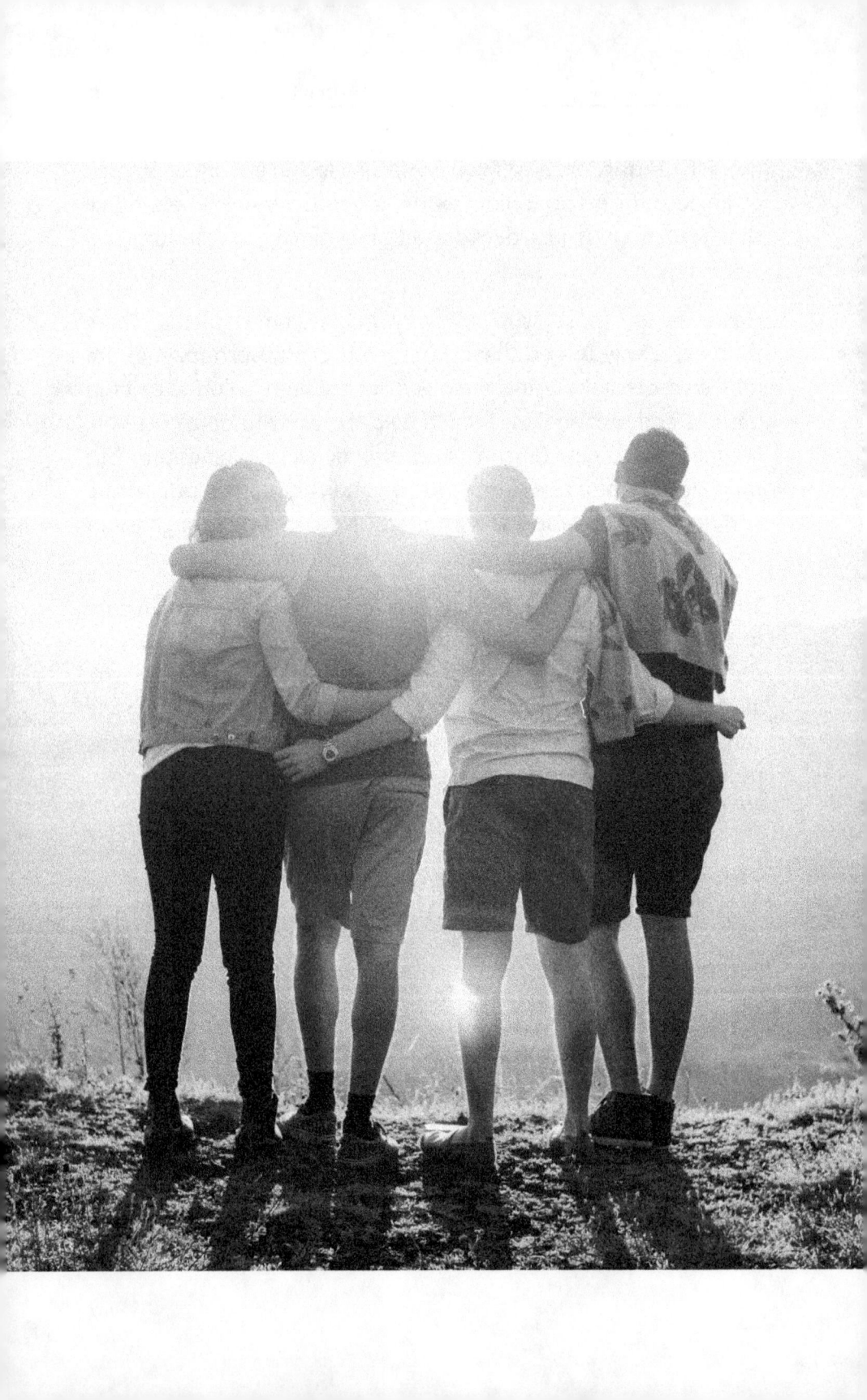

CHAPTER TEN

The Way Out: The First Researched-Backed, Drug-Free PTSD Remedy

Why Everyone Needs an *Energetic System Upgrade*™

Is something missing in your life?

Maybe you can't get along with those close to you...

Or your relationship has lost its spark...

Or your work brings little joy...

Perhaps you're struggling with a health condition...

Or you're secretly jealous of others whose lives—in your mind—are a storybook tale compared to yours.

In reality, when you see beyond the cover stories and masks that everyone shows the world, you discover that millions of people—even those who enjoy worldly success and are surrounded by people who love them—still secretly feel empty.

In the wee hours of the morning, as you lie in bed, you can no longer lie to yourself.

Nor can you escape the harrowing hollowness that cries out to the cosmos: something drastic is missing.

Instead of rising each morning with a sense of joy, excitement and anticipation of the coming day, most people do not face the day with a sense of vibrancy and wondrous anticipation of the miracles that await.

Is this grief due to a missing sense of real purpose or calling in life?

Or is the source of this pain more profound?

And does this pain stem from a deep sense of knowing that your soul is lacking a vital substance that is as central to your survival as air and water?

What is the real source and solution to our epidemic ennui?

At the core, humans crave emotional connection. Being discon-nected from others is the real source of the sorrow that cries out from the deepest depth of our souls; and connecting to others is the cure.

Life on the Earth plane is our love lab.

We are here to learn how to love ourselves and others fully.

And relationships are the stage upon which this laboratory lives.

The highest and most divine purpose of our intimate relationships is to help each other heal what I call the *Old Scars* from childhood. It is these *Old Scars* that block us from fully loving and connecting with others.

My research has proven that the *Old Scars* many carry from their "deformative" years (pun intended) create conflict in adult relation-ships. And much research, including my own, has demonstrated that these relationship conflicts are known to cause HPA-Axis dysfunction. 101, 102 The chemical imbalances associated with

HPA-Axis dysfunction spark the Demand-Withdraw Negative Escalation Cycle, which, in turn, creates a vicious cycle of ever escalating fleeing reactions and intensified relationship conflict. All the fleeing and fighting disconnects—rather than connects—us to those we love.

As we help each other to heal our *Old Scars*, the chemical imbalances and fighting dissipates. Then, and only then, can relationships be mined for the hidden gold—the love and connection that is the buried treasure beneath the mess of *Old Scars*.

Why is mining relationships for healing so elusive to the masses?

For starters, at the deepest level, many of us don't love ourselves as well as we should. The old, negative voices of our parents and significant others buzz in our brains like a swarm of killer bees.

When we enter relationships, especially intimate relationships, we hope that our partners' love will somehow silence these voices and fill the aching, loveless void within.

Rarely does this kind of healing come about.

For two reasons:

First, we unconsciously choose partners who emotionally resemble the people who did us the most harm during our deformative years.

Humans are wired to restage their traumas, again and again reliving the primordial plays of their youth, all in the unconscious hope of finally achieving what I call our *Happy Ending*—the resolution of *Old Scars*.

Tragically, this restaging and reliving rarely brings that *Happy Ending*.

Why?

When we choose partners who are limited and damaged in the exact ways our parents and significant figures of our youth were, we easily fall into repetitions that recreate our earliest disappointments. (Our *Happy Endings* are elusive until we learn how to work with our partners to consciously provide each other with the *Corrective Emotional Experiences* that can heal our *Old Scars*.)

Additionally, because the human mind is programmed to repeat *Old Scars*—rather than guiding our partners to help heal these *Scars*, we behave in ways that induce our partners to act the way the players of our youth did. In this way, our adult relationships repeat our *Old Scars*; and we end up being reinjured rather than repaired.

It has been my life mission to help every living soul break free of these tragic repetitions. My Conflict-Resolution method actually resolves these repetitive patterns and consequent fighting for the majority of those who follow it.

The cornerstone of my method is teaching how to use our intimate relationships to heal our mutual *Old Scars*. As our *Old Scars* heal, fighting and disconnection fade; now, your relationship becomes the soil that seeds your self-love. In turn, your ability to love others grows and grows.

Here is the beauty of this process. As we pour our love onto those closest to us, each intimate relationship becomes a pebble in the proverbial love pond. These reverberations of love have the power to energetically span out to the world, creating world peace and healing the planet one relationship at a time.

When *Old Scars* heal, conflict and fighting fades and intimate relationships become a true source of connection—an endless love song.

Finally, you awaken each day with joyful harmony in your heart, a song that sings out to the world and echoes back into the eternal well of love.

This healing process is what I call the *Energetic System Upgrade*™.

Your *Energetic System Upgrade*™ begins with the application of *Elektra Magnesium*, a transdermal magnesium that I apply to your heart or wherever else I sense is needed. As I've said previously, magnesium is like a biochemical paddle that literally jumpstarts the heart and primes the pump for connection.

Magnesium also helps to reverse the HPA-Axis dysfunction that results from longstanding relationship conflict and fighting. And magnesium quickly switches the internal chemistry from overdrive to peace.

In this peaceful state, you will be ready to embrace what I call *Radical Emotional Nudity*.

It is difficult to impossible to experience true emotional connection without being naked and exposing our deepest selves, while at the same time connecting to the deepest selves of others. This is the only way to cure the disconnection that plagues the world.

One way to be radically emotionally naked is to reveal a painful secret or feeling that has never been spoken aloud.

I know that being this emotionally naked is a frightening prospect for most people.

Why?

Children who are neglected and abused feel that they deserve the mistreatment. This is because children in every country and culture are born with a brain that is ruled by narcissism. (I am the center of the universe and everything that happens around me is about me and because of me). Children's brains are also ruled by omnipotence and magical thinking. (I have the power to change everything around me.)

These thought patterns cause kids to believe:

The abuse and neglect they suffer is their fault. Therefore, they deserve the neglect or mistreatment they are receiving;

And I have the power to change the parent or significant figure who is neglecting and/or mistreating me. When efforts to be a good boy or girl fail to result in better treatment, the child feels like a failure and unlovable.

Most people never get beyond these original thought patterns and behaviors. In adult relationships, many people (especially women) try to be good, hoping to finally earn the love for which they are starving. Of course, this "good girl" pattern doesn't work and creates a greater feeling of disconnection and emptiness.

In order to heal this injury, we must experience what it feels like to be lovable, that is to feel another person loving us to the bottom of our soul.

The only way to be loved at this level is to be vulnerable and radically expose your soul. When you are finally loved at this level, you finally feel you are lovable. This isn't an intellectual exercise. You have to feel the feeling.

Most people never reach the place of self-love because they are too afraid to practice emotional nudity. Precisely because these people believe they are unlovable, they take great pains to not reveal themselves at the deepest core level. Doing so would only bring loathing, right?

Wrong!

Profound healing arises when you have the courage to radically expose your deepest core, *and* these revelations are received with total acceptance and love.

Radical healing is sparked when you feel loved and held, warts and all.

This *Corrective Emotional Experience* provides the unconditional love that we rarely receive as children. It is this holding, acceptance and love of the part of oneself that has been kept hidden that fertilizes the seeds of self-love.

The next step in your **Energetic System Upgrade**™ is learning how to stay in your naked and loving heart when you are hurt and angry.

Intimate relationships are a trigger.

In a nutshell, the unconscious mind constantly links present-day slights with the wounds suffered as a kid. This is what I call the *Emotional Lake Effect.* Think about an actual lake-effect blizzard that gathers moisture and energy as it moves across large expanses of warmer lake water and dumps mounds of snow on the lake's leeward shores. Well, the unconscious mind does the same thing. As the mind dips into the reservoir of the unconscious, it dredges up memories of similar hurts suffered way back when. The next thing you know, you're blowing an emotional gasket because you are reliving all the pain of previous similar offenses. This explains why fireworks go off inside when the current event doesn't seem to warrant such an explosive reaction.

To complicate matters, these associations are happening on an unconscious level, meaning your "feeling memories" are disembodied from the actual events. As a result, it's easy to mistakenly assume that the mountain of emotions you're experiencing is the result of whatever another person just said or did. The next thing you know, you're aiming your broadsides at your partners and friends, family members and colleagues, dumping old emotional baggage onto them without realizing it. This heats the relationship environment to a sizzle and drives those closest to you farther away.

The next task is to focus on how to communicate when you are triggered so that you can guide those closest to you to help heal your *Old Scars*, rather than falling into the trap of camouflaging your pain with anger, which creates the chemical imbalances that cause those closest to you to run away.

Most people, when triggered, dump raw rage on those closest to them, treating those they "love" like emotional toilet bowls. Getting your rocks off on those closest to you is the surest way for your relationships to end up on the rocks. Because relationships are like rubber bands—they can only be stretched so far until they break; and you can't put a rubber band back together. It is important to learn how to think before speaking and only say and do what you know will be helpful to not only yourself but also the other person and the relationship. If you get your rocks off in the moment, you will feel better temporarily. But when you do harm to another, you are ultimately hurting yourself. Whatever you say and do boomerangs back on you.

Humanity must learn to practice what is called impulse control. In order for our world and our relationships to survive and become the source of healing and connection, we must all cultivate impulse control and not lash out when we're triggered.

This is a crucial skill that most of us lack. You will never be able to tap your relationships for healing of self and others if you continue to blast others with your raw rage and push them away.

Next, it's time to learn how to *Identify the Specific Old Scars* that are being triggered inside you by: *Drawing a Fight Map* and *Stripping Away the Overt Content* of the current issue.

Then, it's vital to learn how to talk about your *Old Scars* without attacking the other.

And, to learn how to also communicate what you need to heal (your *Happy Ending*).

And, finally, it's vital to properly listen (which is love in action) when those close to you communicate when they are triggered, so that you can guide them to share what they need to heal their *Old Scars*.

As you use your relationships to heal your mutual *Old Scars*, anger and fighting disappear. Then, your thirsty heart can be quenched as you drink from the well of love that brought you together. It is this eternally flowing well of love that extinguishes the flames that burn most relationships, families and countries. It is this same well that keeps the love fires burning eternally, so that you may live the ultimate truth: Love Never Dies.

I invite you to become a pebble in the proverbial love pond by experiencing your own **Energetic System Upgrade**.

To celebrate the launch of this book, I am offering a limited number of **Energetic System Upgrade** sessions at a great discount. To find out more and to schedule, visit: DrJamieTurndorf.com/EnergeticSystemUpgrade

Here are Some Unsolicited Testimonials for the first **Energetic System Upgrade** Workshop at 1440 Multiversity:

"Hi Jamie, The week end at 1440 with that group was amazing! I am still reeling from it in a good way. Many insights and dreams keep flooding my being. I am also listening to your book, *Love Never Dies*, and allowing a new way of looking at those who have left their body to settle in my psyche. Any fear of dying that I had seems to be gone, knowing that my consciousness just moves on to another realm.

The only survey I received from 1440 was about the facility itself and very little detail on the programming, although I did rate those at the highest level. Thank you!

I will continue to follow you on social media and will look for any future groups to participate in. Much Love,"

-- Karen

"I took the survey from 1440 and gave you a well-deserved excellent review. The workshop was more than I imagined and, as long as I practice what I learned -- which I have been doing -- I know that I will only get better. My ego thanks you and so does my soul! Our local junior college has creative writing classes and I intend to sign up, so there's progress already.

I would be interested in learning more about the online groups, so please send me information. Thanks again for upgrading my electrical system. It needed it. After the class, I bought your book, *Love Never Dies*. Can't wait to read it.

Love,"

-- Carol

"Hi Jamie, Thank you for sharing your healing wisdom and energy with our group at 1440. It was deep and powerful, even profound. I love your humor and your energy, and that you are grounded in real psychology as well as spirituality. Many thanks,"

-- Kacey

"Dear Jamie, Our meeting and healing sessions at 1440 were transformational. I feel so blessed and grateful for the wisdom teaching that I was skillfully guided to receive by yourself. Recognizing, feeling and then healing a core wound and faulty belief system continues to be so huge for me. I have shared my experiences with you with my husband and a few close friends that I know will benefit. Thank you again,"

-- Rebecca

"Hello Jamie, I am forever grateful for such an amazing experience. Your truly a special healer and felt a great connection to the others in the group as well.

I believe your workshop was the beginning of my awakening. The tools I left will provide me with great comfort and skills to continue working on my purpose. When you touched on the magnesium deficiency I was moved having been suffering from so many ailments, seeking out so many Dr's being given pill after pill after pill with a revolving vicious cycle of physical, mental, and emotional pain with no clarity I believe I finally got the diagnosis I wish I would have gotten 25 years ago.

I want to thank you wholeheartedly from the bottom of my heart for having the opportunity to be able to connect and impact people in the way that you do. Your work truly touched and changed me as an individual but also as a group. I am forever grateful for such a transforming healing experience.

With Love,"

--Jen J

These Testimonials are from the 1440 Multiversity Online *Energetic System Upgrade*™ Workshop:

Hi Jamie,

I feel like I held down the rage towards my mom. But also in a way I didn't feel like I had to perform either so that might've been

119

growth as well. I still feel it (like a lump right at the bottom of my throat/top of my chest). I didn't feel ready to let'r rip like Dan did or I did that time a few weeks ago with you in group. It's ok I know and I have next group or session. I feel like seeing my mom in this light my still be somewhat new for me and am processing.

I thought that the retreat/seminar was incredible and there was a wonderful energy about the group and all of the participants. You were great, open and your usual knowledgable self, guiding everyone through the experience. I would love to do it again! It was like a new group for me but everyone was already primed and ready to jump in the deep end!

Big love and XX,

--T

Tim's additional growth:

This was such an amazing group. I realized that my sovereignty and my power will come from truly feeling the absolute disappointment and injustice of never getting what I needed from my mother. But my salvation will be in acknowledging that my mother as I knew her never was. She was never there in the way that I needed her to be. She was limited and hobbled in her emotional capacity. My rage towards her is my weakness. My sadness is my strength. My courage to be with my sadness is my strength. This makes sense because I didn't have the strength to be with my sadness until now and this is why I have been in a vicious cycle. Jamie, seeing you take your power and baptizing yourself with your own tears in the Mediterranean was so powerful to me. It was such a demonstration of resolve, willpower, strength, self determination and sovereignty. I internalized this image for myself. I do have the strength to be with the sadness and mourning of my mother. I want to differentiate from my Mother/Father. My courage to be

120

with this tremendous and heavy sadness is how outwardly and inwardly I can show Little Tim how 'we' are doing things differently; how we are taking a different path and separating, not out of desperate and impotent rage but out of true and deep understanding of the sadness and recognition of what I never had in the first place. I WILL ALLOW MYSELF TO FEEL THIS SADNESS.

I love you.

--T

I am grateful as well for the breakthrough I experienced regarding long-suppressed thoughts and emotions. It's very unusual for me to share such intimate feelings with a new group and I truly appreciate the receptivity and support that everyone provided.

I look forward to our next get together.

That was a very powerful and energizing session. Being able to share the abusive social experience in a group setting I think was much more empowering than if I was just to share it in on 1-1 session. Thank you for assembling such a varied and intuitive group.

--Dan

Dan's Continued Healing:

Jamie - as it's been two weeks since the Energetic System Upgrade I thought I'd check in with you and the group to share a couple of observations I've had that relate to my breakthrough during the session. First, I acted on the guidance you shared in our one on one session immediately following the group regarding using my new found courage to step directly into the line of my wife's fury when it arises and to listen with compassion for the deeper meaning behind her anger instead of trying to combat it or avoid it. This new approach has impacted both of us. For me it is uncovering a new stronger identity, one that is grounded in emotion and more genuinely masculine and mature than before. For Kelly, I've noticed her anger dissipating more quickly than in the past and seen her start to ask for things she wants in a more direct way- like last night when she asked me simply if I wanted to go with her on a walk instead of asking with a demanding tone or just heading out on her own.

Standing in strength is also changing the dynamic that exists between us and our children. Before, I think I was expecting Kelly to parent me in a way and used to always side with the kids when it came to indulgences like sweets. I've started to exert my own authority in parenting our girls, however, and as such believe I'm taking some of the burden off of her. The result is that Kelly has softened, our kids aren't running quite as rampantly around the house as they were before, and there's a growing tone of calm and quiet that we haven't had in our house for a long time.

I think it's also important to share that this practice of standing tall in the face of fury has not been exactly easy. At first it felt like a leap of faith where I lead with my heart and hoped that whatever outward appearance I was wearing would be sufficiently convincing to overcome the long standing dynamic of conflict between us. But I'm gaining confidence with every encounter and anticipate that this way of showing up will become more and more natural over time.

Thanks again to you and the group for your support during that amazing session. I hope we all get the chance to meet again before too long.

--Dan

Hello Jamie,

Thank you for the invitation to the Energetic System Upgrade workshop.

It was incredible. It helped me so much. I was able to start the process of facing the man that fathered me. To be able to start getting past the guilt trip he put on me as a young child. Even though I am not ready to accept an apology from him, I feel so much better, healthier and stronger.

I am also grateful to have had the opportunity to meet new people who are also struggling with life situations because of traumatic experiences in the their past. I was able to relate and feel their pain as well. It was a connection that I will never forget.

The 4 hours went by so quickly. A regroup meeting sounds like a plan.

Please feel free to share my comments with the rest of the group.

With deep gratitude and best regards.

--Kathy

Hi Jamie,

Thank you very much for our Energetic System Upgrade call! I am so glad you encouraged me to attend. As you predicted, I related to everyone's experience.

It was amazing to discover that there was a part of my story in something that each person shared. I've learned more about the belief (that I have) that the people I love leave me because something is inherently wrong with me. I learned more about my fear of abandonment. Also about my guilt for my murderous rage towards my mother and even my ex-husband's rage towards his mother turned into me. Wow! I believe we all felt connected and that no one wanted to leave the call! What an amazing gift of healing. I'm savoring the feelings now. Thank you.

Thank you all! What an eye-opener and a day of healing it was for me. Having related to everything that I did, it helped me to realize the impact being an Empath has had on my life. I also related to, and acknowledged my own "playing it small" to avoid jealousy/being hated. I forgot to mention that in my summary. You wouldn't know it by how freely I shared, but I normally avoid groups! I consider it fate that we were together. I really would like to meet again.

Have a wonderful week!

In deep gratitude.

Much love,

--Dee

Dr Jamie,

Thank you yet again. Our one on one session years ago shifted and healed a grief in me that I'd been carrying just below the surface since I was 10 years old, and it hasn't come back. Now my 2nd group session, both equally powerful.

This group was a great experience, amazing how easily we were all able to connect. Fantastic to see how everyone shifted within the session. Lovely to get and share feedback.

I went into the workshop frustrated at not taking care of myself as much as I support and help others, basically (unnecessarily) neglecting myself.

My work is Rapid Transformational Therapy, and now I've decided to treat myself like I do my clients/friends/family, I'm giving myself that attention for the very first time. Oy!

The similarity we shared, that we are all still profoundly affected by a childhood treatment, made me think that it's time to let go, it really doesn't serve any purpose for me anymore. There were things that definitely weren't right, but somehow I'm here, miraculously survived it all, as we all did, it could have been better (should have been better!) but, what the heck, I'm here now.

After the session I fell asleep - and slept for hours!!! Anyone else? Definitely more relaxed, I've taken the pressure off myself.

Thank you all, best wishes,

--Suzanne

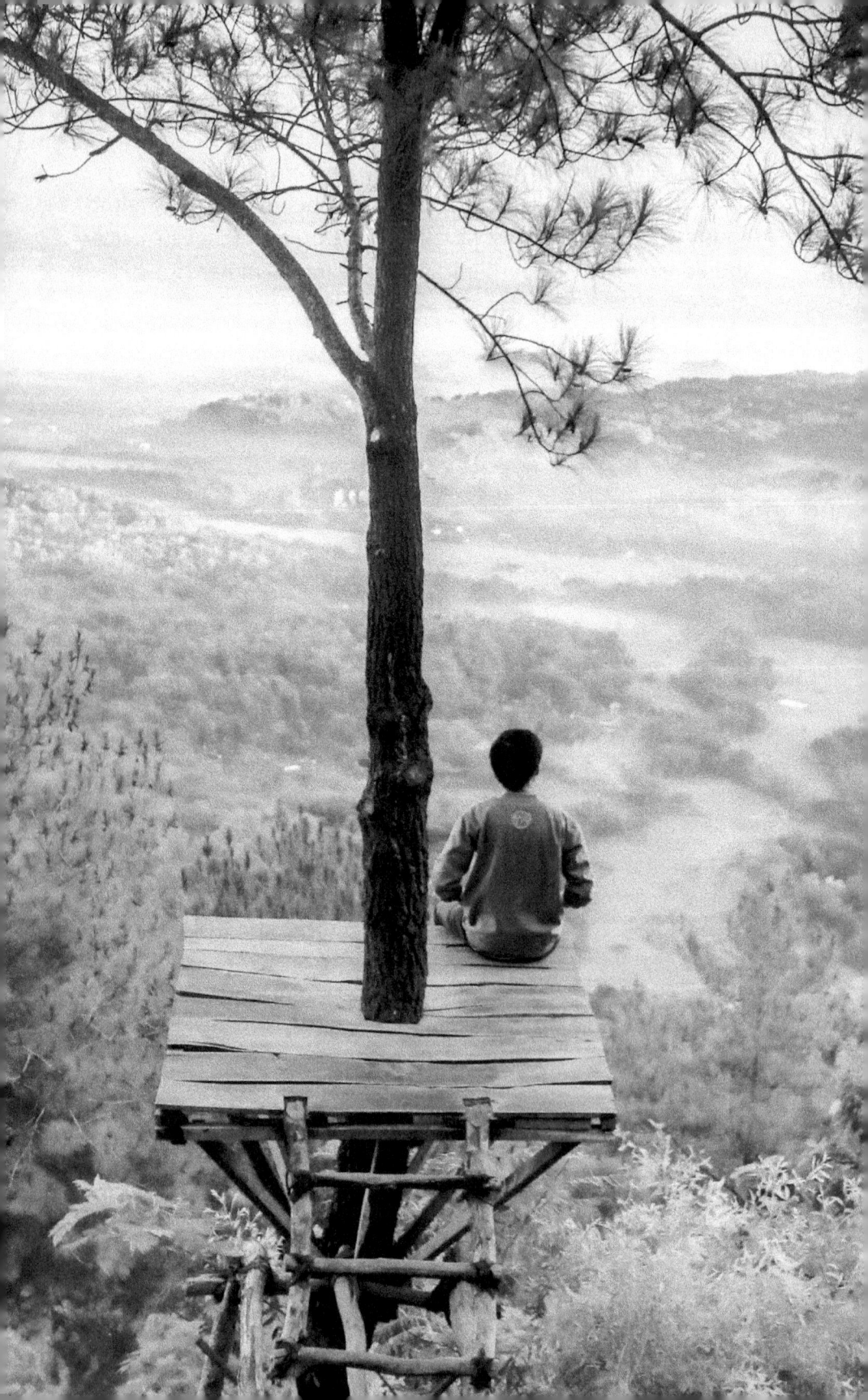

Conclusion

In this book, I have provided scientific evidence linking stress with cellular depletion of magnesium. I have also shown the evidence that magnesium depletion triggers PTSD (and many other conditions and diseases, as well). Finally, I have provided research demonstrating that supplementing with magnesium—especially transdermal magnesium, the most absorbable form—remedies PTSD and over 100 conditions and diseases that result from deficiency of this major mineral.

It's important to note that stress comes in many forms, including physical, biochemical, emotional and spiritual.

As you know, the mind, body, and our emotions are truly one entity; we cannot separate one part of ourselves from the other.

What's more, we know that emotions cause chemical and bodily (physical and biochemical) stress.

When we speak of stress, we're actually referring to a term that encompasses the deeper emotion called fear.

We fear the loss of a loved one; we fear loss of our income; we fear for our health and for the health of our loved ones…

When we peel back the psychological onion layers of fear, we uncover the universal fear of death.

When my beloved husband of nearly 30 years, Emile Jean Pin (who I mentioned previously was a world-renowned former Jesuit priest who the Dalai Lama named as one of the 50 men of all time who was one with God) left his body from a bee sting, he began proving his presence through astonishing manifestations. These manifestations are not only meant for me; they are meant to let you know that we don't die; we just leave our bodies.

As a result of Jean's cataclysmic proof of soul survival, I also realized that our relationships are not meant to end with bodily death. When we form a bond with another soul, that bond is eternal. We are not meant to be separated. I say this to remind you that your loved ones in spirit are right here and waiting to reconnect and stay connected to you.

My reminding you of this truth will, I hope, assist in alleviating any residual terror of "death" and "dying."

When we are freed of the fear of our own demise or the bodily loss of those we love, we can then address the most important question of our existence:

Why are we here?

As I said previously, Earth is our Love Lab.

Our only purpose on Earth is to perfect our ability to love ourselves and others.

And our intimate relationships are the stage upon which we are invited to perfect our performances.

What consists of an ideal performance?

For starters, all evolved souls are being asked to live the profound duality that consists of shedding the fear of "death" and "dying" while concurrently living each day as though it may be our last.

If you knew today were to be your last day on Earth, how would you behave differently with those closest to you?

First, I would have you begin by eulogizing the living. By this I mean tell those close to you what you love about them and why. And, remember to do this daily.

Next, I would ask you to remember that in order to live love now, you must perfect your ability to manage your raw, negative impulses. By this I refer to managing the angry feelings that are triggered whenever our psychological toes are stepped on. Our natural default is to camouflage our boo boos with anger. Most people act on the anger by lashing out at those they love most.

Love cannot thrive when anger and fighting predominates. Sadly, most people do not know how to manage the inevitable conflicts that arise in our intimate relationships. And the real reason most relationships fall apart is not because of inadequate love but rather because our love is eroded by unresolved conflicts and the angry feelings that go with it. Most people act out their anger using what I call *Open* and *Secret Warfare Fight Traps*, which include yelling, screaming, delivering paybacks and putdowns. These *Fight Traps* ultimately rupture our relationships and destroy love.

As I've said previously: While it feels good in the moment to get your rocks off on another person, on the rocks is where your relationships will end up if you don't manage your mouth and your actions. Remember, whatever you say and do boomerangs back on you. If you hurt another person, you are ultimately hurting yourself.

I have spent my entire 37-year career researching and developing methods for heading-off and resolving the inevitable conflicts that arise in our intimate relationships. I've written many books in which I've presented my Conflict-Resolution method.

Heading off-fights and resolving conflicts boils down to this: We all need to pull up our big boy and big girl pants and grow up. Growing up means we are not allowed to dump verbal turds on one another. Or engage in damaging actions against another.

This is easier said than done, I know.

Our world is in great turmoil now.

We are being quarantined in close quarters. It's easy to get on each other's last nerves.

But beyond the current state of affairs, there's a deeper reason why those closest to us trigger our anger.

Strong angry feelings are a clue that unfinished business lurks beneath the surface of our fights. It goes without saying that each time you fight the same fight and lose, you are more aggravated than the time before. But there is another reason for the intensity of your reactions. In a nutshell, our unconscious minds constantly link present day slights with the wounds we suffered as kids. I again refer to what I call the *Emotional Lake Effect*, which is akin to the actual Lake Effect in which a storm gathers moisture and force in its sweep across the Great Lakes. As I said previously, the unconscious mind does the exact same thing. As the mind dips into the reservoir of our unconscious, it dredges up memories of similar hurts that we suffered as kids. The next thing you know, you're blowing an emotional gasket because you are literally reliving all the pain of previous similar offenses. This explains why fireworks are going off inside you even though the current event doesn't seem to warrant such an explosive reaction.

To complicate matters, these associations are happening on an unconscious level, meaning your "feeling memories" are disembodied from the actual events. As a result, it's easy to mistakenly assume that the mountain of emotions you're experiencing is the result of whatever those close to you just said or did. The next thing you know, you're aiming your cannons at the other person, and dumping old emotional baggage onto them without realizing it. This heats the climate to a sizzle.

During this precious time at home, I encourage you to perfect your performance:

Turn down the emotional thermostat when your internal temperature starts to rise.

Vow to keep a civil tongue in your mouth rather than deliver a tongue-lashing.

Walk away when you're triggered. Splash water on your face, and calm down.

When alone, identify the deepest layer of what triggered your anger. This means going back in your memory and uncovering the *Old Scar* that lurks beneath the current event, which is just a smokescreen. I call this process "Stripping" and, no, I'm not talking about getting "naked!" I'm talking about stripping away the overt, here-and-now fight content to uncover the real issue, the *Old Scar*, that's been triggered. (I fully outline how to *Strip Away the Overt Content to Uncover the Old Scar that Lurks Beneath* in Kiss Your Fights Goodbye.)

Next, calmly speak to the person who triggered you about what's really going on for you.

To ensure that you receive the gift of being heard, it's vital to present a message that's hearable (Say no to *Open* or *Secret Warfare Fight Traps*, which include name-calling, character assassination, guilt-tripping, etc. I fully outline all the dysfunctional *Fight Traps* in Kiss

Your Fights Goodbye. If you want love to thrive, it's necessary to identify and eliminate all your *Fight Traps*.)

When you speak, use my X/Y Formula and simply describe in a calm way what was said or done (that's X) and how you feel about it (that's Y). Reformulate the sentence so the word "you" is omitted. Instead of saying, "I feel X when YOU say or do Y" say instead, "I feel X when Y is said or done."

Most importantly, when describing what was said or done and how you feel, you must mention the *Old Scar* that was activated by the current trigger. In this way, you are mining your intimate relationships for their highest and most divine purpose—to help each other heal our *Old Scars* from childhood. In discussing your *Old Scar*, you instantly transform the person who stepped on your psychological toes from enemy into ally, enabling him or her to empathize with your early pain, and give you the response you needed way back when. In this way, we help each other heal our *Old Scars*. As the *Old Scars* are healed, anger and fighting fade away.

As a final note, on the road to conflict resolution, listening is the superhighway.

Ninety-nine percent of conflicts can be resolved by truly listening and understanding each other.

This is because listening is love in action.

Keep in mind that listening is an active process of conveying that we heard what the presenter is saying. We do this by repeating back what we heard and allowing the presenter to correct our understanding until the presenter says, "You got it."

Good listening is so powerful because it provides the deepest healing of our *Old Scars*. As we listen with love, we offer what's called the corrective emotional experience, as we understand each other's pain the way many of our parents may not have done.

God gave us two ears and one mouth so we would listen more and speak less.

I invite you to transform your house into a true love lab.

The essential ingredient in your lab is transdermal magnesium, which I call the "love mineral." This is because magnesium acts like a biochemical paddle that electromagnetically jumpstarts the brain and the heart, creating an instant shift from stress to chemical balance and calm. Being in an open and receptive state enables you to absorb new ways of handling conflicts, and keeping anger at bay, thereby allowing you to fully embrace the divine call to love.

APPENDIX
PTSD Scientific Fact Sheet

According to the NIH, 44 million Americans including 5.5-6 million veterans reported struggling with PTSD as of June 2019. That is the tip of the iceberg because most people don't know they have PTSD and don't receive treatment.

The epidemiological studies and controlled trials confirm that most of us are at least moderately deficient in magnesium.[103]

Stress (emotional, biochemical and/or environmental) causes a rapid and massive depletion of magnesium from the body.[104]

Magnesium depletion triggers a chemical imbalance called HPA-Axis dysfunction.[105]

HPA-Axis dysfunction causes PTSD.[106]

Magnesium supplementation reverses PTSD.[107]

One accident, illness or trauma is sufficient to trigger PTSD.

Magnesium is an essential nutrient needed in over 1000 bodily functions.

Nearly every disease is a magnesium deficiency in disguise.

Impure water, processed foods, refined sugar and carbs, alcohol, soda, certain foods such as tannins from black and green tea, phytic acid from unfermented soy products and unsoaked grains and seeds, oxalic acid from raw spinach, coffee, smoking, GMOs, gluten, damaged fats/oils, fluoride toxicity and other neurotoxins and endotoxins, pharmaceutical drugs (especially diuretics, bronchodilators such as theophylline for asthma, birth control pills, insulin, beta blockers, digitalis, tetracycline and some other antibiotics, corticosteroids, antipsychotics and cocaine) toxic metals such as mercury, lead and aluminum, pesticides and herbicides such as glyphosate residues in our food and water results in our becoming depleted of magnesium.

Our Western diet and lifestyle results in nearly every person being deficient in magnesium—meaning everyone has some degree of PTSD.

Magnesium deficiency worsens with age, which explains why people become sicker, less stress tolerant and more and more prone to PTSD as we grow older.

The stress of COVID-19 has pushed our magnesium deficient world over the edge, triggering a *Global PTSD Pandemic Stress Syndrome* epidemic.

Oral magnesium causes diarrhea and gastrointestinal symptoms at worst, and 30% absorption, at best.[108]

Transdermal magnesium provides superior cellular absorption. This study compared low dose oral magnesium versus transdermal administration. Urinary levels were tested and demonstrated transdermal administration provided better absorption than oral administration.[109, 110, 111, 112]

MAGNESIUM QUESTIONS AND ANSWERS

If my doctor tells me my blood test shows I have normal magnesium levels, doesn't that mean I am not deficient?

Answer: No!

Beware of the mainstream misconceptions regarding the use of blood tests for detecting magnesium deficiency. Even Healthline. com erroneously says,

"The symptoms of magnesium deficiency are usually subtle unless your levels become severely low. Deficiency may cause fatigue, muscle cramps, mental problems, irregular heartbeat and osteoporosis. If you believe you may have a magnesium deficiency, your suspicions can be confirmed with a simple blood test."

Most doctors are not aware of research proving that serum (blood) tests are not an accurate measure of magnesium levels. The NIH site says regarding Mg status testing: "No single method is considered satisfactory."[113]

You can't test accurately for magnesium deficiency because the blood levels are kept relatively normal, despite the tissue cell levels (where 99% of your Mg resides) being low. Because the body needs to maintain a very specific level of magnesium (in a very narrow range) in the bloodstream in order for the heart to continue beating, in order to keep blood levels high enough, the body pulls magnesium from the organs and cells, causing undetected cellular low magnesium.

Hence, blood tests are not accurate indicators of magnesium status. Best indicators are the symptomology. Hair analysis is only a general guide because the status is usually about 6 months out of date (depending on the length of hair that is cut for analysis). Then we depend on knowing exactly the right balance of the minerals, and we still don't know from this test about any magnesium-blocking agents like glyphosate or other chemical toxins that may be present. So even hair analysis is just a guide.

If you have low magnesium symptoms and you supply transdermal magnesium and the symptoms dissipate, isn't that a sufficient test?

Is there a more accurate way to test my magnesium levels?

Answer:

There are two ways to test cellular magnesium levels: 1) Hair analysis, which is a long-term blueprint of body chemistry, is a better way to test magnesium levels; and 2) In addition to hair analysis, which is a non-invasive way to test long-term magnesium levels and ratios, the Exatest (http://exatest.com/Research.htm) is an oral cheek swab, which provides an accurate current measure of intracellular magnesium levels. If you're working with an alternative or open-minded doctor, you can request that he/she order this test for you.

Can you overdose on magnesium?

Answer:

In the Western world we're programmed to think in terms of drugs and dosing, and dangers of over-dosing. This paradigm doesn't apply to transdermal magnesium chloride salt, which is nutrition via skin. Think of the tissues and cells of your body as your magnesium storage tank. The body holds the nutrients inside the epidermal reservoir and draws on them gradually from this reservoir as needed. The body is in control with this system. The tank needs to be full at all times so that your body can pull from these stores in times of sickness and stress. Keeping a full tank is a preemptive operation that heads off deficiency. Magnesium ions are stored in the cell membrane as Mg-ATP, like storage batteries in reserve. What still needs to be exposed is how important choles-terol fats are to cell functions. For so long cholesterol has been demonized. Yet the integrity of the cell wall depends on a lipid bi-layer structure held together by the charge of magnesium ions. The body is so hungry for magnesium (in the right absorbable salt form) that it can't have enough reserves of magnesium!

The NIH site says toxicity can result at over 5,000 mg per day <u>oral</u> supplement. Note: It's impossible to get this much transdermally. Very large doses of magnesium-containing laxatives and antacids (typically providing more than 5,000 mg/day magnesium) have been associated with magnesium toxicity. Symptoms of magnesium toxicity usually develop after serum concentrations exceed 1.74–2.61 mmol/L.

According to Dr. Sircus, "Risk of magnesium toxicity is usually related to severe renal insufficiency-when the kidney loses the ability to remove excess magnesium. Individuals with impaired kidney function are at a higher risk for adverse effects from magnesium supplementation." Because kidney problems indicate magnesium deficiency, Dr. Sircus recommends transdermal magnesium absorption as the safest way for those with renal issues to access magnesium, by starting with a low dose application and adjusting as needed over time. In *Transdermal Magnesium Therapy: A New Modality for the Maintenance of Health*, Sircus provides medical dose information for doctors treating chron-ically ill patients.[114]

Despite more than 20 years of popular use of magnesium bathing, magnesium oils, creams and lotions, there is as yet no evidence in the scientific literature indicating topical magnesium can cause hypermagnesemia (magnesium excess in the cells).

So, to answer the question, can you OD on transdermal magnesium? Highly unlikely and nearly impossible! If you use one all-over application of Magnesium Cream (2 tsp) that's only 300 mg magnesium. If you add on one teaspoon of Magnesium Lotion, that's another 300 mg. If you add on 6 sprays of Magnesium Oil Spritz that's another 300 mg. If you do all of these things, you are still only reaching 900-1,000 magnesium applied to skin. The epidermis stores the nutrients as a reservoir which the body draws from moderately over time. It can take several hours before all of the available magnesium is finally taken up by the body, because it is only drawing in according to requirements due to our homeostatic systems. It doesn't all go in at once quickly. The body takes in only what it can utilize at any one time. It is a gradual, sustainable uptake. See the study links regarding transdermal magnesium here:[115]

The real danger is not in getting too much magnesium, but not getting enough of it!

Is transdermal magnesium safe for children and pregnant women?

Answer:

Yes, this form of magnesium is safe also for little children and pregnant women.

Can't I just take an oral magnesium supplement?

Answer:

If you are not overly deficient in magnesium, then a 30% uptake plus dietary magnesium and not too much stress may be enough.

The most common magnesium supplement you will find in stores is magnesium oxide because it's the cheapest, but only 4% bioavailable according to the studies because this compound is very insoluble for cells as the body first needs to break down and reform the magnesium so it joins up with two chlorine ions and becomes magnesium chloride.

The citrate version is a bit better.

The most absorbable forms of oral magnesium are magnesium glycinate, fumarate or orotate. Even the most absorbable forms of magnesium result in a 30% absorption rate at best.

Magnesium chloride is the most common form of magnesium salt derived from sea water, and the most bio-available because it is very water soluble and able to access cells without further digestion required. Chloride ions are also the most abundant of the negatively charged ions used by the body. We need a lot of it! Therefore, the body hungrily takes it up. As soon as magnesium chloride is dissolved and diluted it is easily absorbed by cells— including skin cells—as in magnesium soaking (great for detox and sleep). When we infuse magnesium chloride with plant fats it is even more readily absorbed by skin because skin is lipophilic (loves fats). The fats of the **Elektra Magnesium** cream and lotion hold magnesium ions inside the epidermis like food in a smorgasbord. The skin has a large reservoir storage potential when juicy fats are available to hold moisture in. This system beats tablets hands down! Transdermal magnesium also works much faster because it bypasses the digestive system. Magnesium not only transits in blood, but has been shown in studies to also be able to pass between tissue cells.

The more expensive magnesium compounds sold as tablets are a chelated magnesium (ie. magnesium joined up with amino acids of some kind like magnesium taurate, magnesium glycinate, fumarate, etc.) and they do offer benefits because people can be deficient in the other compounded nutrient. But there is a limit as to how much magnesium can be digested and absorbed through the bowel wall, into the bloodstream and eventually into our tissue cells. The bowel wall is sensitive and seems to optimally absorb only the low concentration that would be naturally occurring in spring waters or foods. Studies show that as researchers incrementally increased the concentration of the magnesium in the drinking water, there was a corresponding inverse relationship with uptake of magnesium. That is, the higher the concentration, the more the excess ends up being expelled by the digestive system. [116, 117]

In his book *Transdermal Magnesium Therapy*, Sircus said that even the best quality practitioner magnesium oral tablet supplements (a chelated magnesium with amino acid) aren't absorbed more than 40% at best. So, the majority of oral magnesium supplements are lost in the stool. There are just too many digestion issues with tablets, especially if you don't have enough stomach acid to break up the magnesium compound. Magnesium chelate (bound with an amino acid) is less likely to cause diarrhea, but that is not an indicator of cell absorption, which requires the magnesium to be combined as a chloride compound to be fully water soluble and able to be taken up by cells.

Absorbability of the magnesium in tablets also diminishes the higher the magnesium dose at one time. If you keep taking increasing amounts it will liquefy stool and almost all comes out too fast.

After magnesium passes through the stomach, you have to be able to get it through the bowel wall, and that presents another obstacle. Optimal absorption of magnesium via gut wall is achieved only with lower concentrations, such as what would be in natural spring waters or foods. As we increase magnesium concentration, there is a curvilinear reduction in uptake, i.e. less uptake the higher the concentration.

This is nowhere near enough for high end magnesium needs. Transdermal magnesium offers a larger storage reservoir in the skin, and can deliver more magnesium in the right form for cellular uptake; and in a sustained release manner because the body is in control of uptake as is needed, drawing in only what can be utilized at any one time.

I'm using transdermal magnesium. So why am I not seeing results or improvement in my condition?

Answer:

Some people experience a faster effect than others.

In cases of great magnesium deficiency, there just isn't enough to go around to make noticeable headway to compensate for the greater load of stored wastes and toxins (which create an acidic cell environment). It's not so much about getting magnesium into the cell (which happens easily with magnesium chloride, but not so easily with oral forms of magnesium supplement), as much as getting enough magnesium over time to make a compensatory difference for the stored wastes and toxins. This is why also working from the other end with diet and cleansing strategies helps lighten the workload of magnesium and leverage its effects. Two ends towards the middle.

Also, many people are too timid with it in the beginning (not using enough), which means a much longer time for symptoms and conditions to resolve.

If you're frustrated with your progress on the transdermal magnesium, you may be a "magnesium waster" meaning your body flushes a lot of it out. In which case, double the dose!

Can magnesium protect me against environmental chemicals, such as fluoride and glyphosate?

Answer:

We absorb fluorides and glyphosate from various sources without knowing it. For example, even if we don't drink fluoridated tap water, but still drink some other kind of beverage made with fluoridated water, we still ingest nearly the same amount of fluoride. Even a common orange juice that supermarkets sell has 0.7 ppm fluoride (water supply in Australia is dosed to 1ppm). Fluorides can also outgas from Teflon, fabric coatings, and fire retardants, and can also be ingested via pharmaceuticals. It is mind-blowing how many potential exposures for fluoride there are.

Likewise, even if we eat an organic diet, we can't fully avoid exposure and ingestion of glyphosate. This is because organic farmers use conventional manure, which contains glyphosate. The glyphosate in the manure ends up in organic foods. In addition, acid rain exposes us to glyphosate residues from gardens thousands of miles away.

But we can protect against inadvertent ingestion of these poisons using extra transdermal magnesium, because magnesium binds to fluoride and glyphosate, transforming these chemicals into water-soluble substances than can be easily excreted.

Could my low thyroid be linked to chemical exposure combined with low magnesium?

Answer:

Chemicals like fluorides, glyphosate, pthalates, plastics and xenoestrogens (like soy products) can disrupt thyroid function along with lack of iodine, magnesium, selenium and L-tyrosine. If more chemicals are absorbed that block our digestion or nutrient uptake, we tend to need more of the nutrients to compensate and defend. Avoiding the chemicals and increasing nutrient density gives us the best shot at thyroid health.

Where Can I Buy Elektra Magnesium?

Answer: You can purchase **Elektra Magnesium** directly from the manufacturer: http://www.elektramagnesium.com.au

The world's first natural magnesium cream:

- Natural (chem-free)
- GMO Free
- Glyphosate Free
- Fair trade shea butter
- Re-used & recycled packaging
- Australian made
- Vegan friendly

End Notes

Foreword

1 Galland L., MD. (1991-1992). *Magnesium Trace Elements.* "Magnesium, stress and neuropsychiatric disorders" 10(2-4):287-301.

2 Adshead, G. (August 2000). *The British Journal of Psychiatry.* "Psychological therapies for posttraumatic stress disorder" Volume 177, Issue 2, 144-148.

3 Dunlop, B. W., Wong, A. (March 2019). *Progress in Neuro-Psychopharmacology & Biological Psychiatry.* "The hypothalamic-pituitary-adrenal axis in PTSD: Pathophysiology and treatment interventions" 8;89:361-379.

4 Sartori, S. B., Whittle, N. [...], and Singewald, N. (January 2012).

Neuropharmacology. "Magnesium deficiency induces anxiety and HPA axis dysregulation: Modulation by therapeutic drug treatment" Volume 62, Issue 1, 304-312.

5 Fulop, T., MD, PhD, FACP, FASN, Chief Editor, and Batuman V., MD, FASN. (Oct 30, 2020). *Medscape.com.* "How is magnesium absorbed?"

6 Kass, L., Rosanoff, A. [...], and Plesset, M. (2017). *PLOS ONE.* "Effect of transdermal magnesium cream on serum and urinary magnesium levels in humans: A pilot study" 12(4); e0174817.

7 Seeling, M. (October 1994). *Journal of the American College of Nutrition.* "Consequences of magnesium deficiency on the enhancement of stress reactions: Preventive and therapeutic implications (A review)" 13(5):429-46.

Introduction

8 Dean, C., MD, ND. (2006). *The Magnesium Miracle* (Revised and Updated Edition). New York: Ballantine Books.

9 No authors listed. (9/17/2019). *RxList.com.* "Magnesium"

Chapter One

10 Gradus, J., L., DSc, MPH. (no date). *VA US Department of Veterans Affairs (PTSD.VA.GOV) PTSD: National Center for PTSD.* "Epidemiology of PTSD" https://www.ptsd.va.gov/professional/treat/essentials/epidemiology.asp.

11 Adshead, G. (August 2000). *The British Journal of Psychiatry.* "Psychological therapies for posttraumatic stress disorder" Volume 177, Issue 2, 144-148.

12 Sherin, J. E., MD, PhD and Nemeroff, C.B., MD, PhD, (September 13, **2011**). *Dialogues Clinical Neuroscience.* "Post-traumatic stress disorder: the neurobiological impact of psychological trauma" September 13(3) 2011, 263-278.

13 No authors listed. (no date). *Anxiety and Depression Association of America (ADAA.org).* "Symptoms of PTSD" https://adaa.org/understanding-anxiety/posttraumatic-stress-disorder-ptsd/symptoms.

14 Sartori, S. B., and Whittle, N. [...], and Singewald, N. (January 2012).

Neuropharmacology. "Magnesium deficiency induces anxiety and HPA axis dysregulation: Modulation by therapeutic drug treatment" Volume 62, Issue 1, 304-312.

Chapter Two

15 No authors listed. (no date). *VA US Department of Veterans Affairs (PTSD.VA.GOV) PTSD: National Center for PTSD.* "How Common is PTSD in Women?"

https://www.ptsd.va.gov/understand/common/common_women.asp.

16 Irish, L. A., Fischer, B., Fallon, W., Spoonster, E., Sledjeski, E., M., and Delahanty, D. L. (March 2011). *Journal of Anxiety Disorders.* "Gender Differences in PTSD Symptoms: An Exploration of Peritraumatic Mechanisms" 25(2): 209-216.

17 Christiansen, D. M., and Hansen, M. (2015). *European Journal of Psychotraumatology.* "Accounting for sex differences in PTSD: A multi-variable mediation model" 6, 26068. doi:10.3402/ejpt.v6.26068.

18 Friling J. L. (2017). *European Journal of Psychotraumatology.* "Preventing PTSD with oxytocin: Effects of oxytocin administration on fear neurocircuitry and PTSD symptom development in recently trauma-exposed individuals" 8(1), 1302652. doi:10.1080/20008198.2017.1302652.

19 Ford, V. (August 21, 2019). *Successtms.com.* *"How PTSD Symptoms are Different in Women than Symptoms in Men"* https://successtms.com/blog/ptsd-symptoms-in-women-vs-men.

20 No authors listed. (Oct 31, 2014). *Ottawa (ON): Canadian Agency for Drugs and Technologies in Health. CADTH Rapid Response Reports.* "Transcranial Magnetic Stimulation for the

Treatment of Adults with PTSD, GAD, or Depression: A Review of Clinical Effectiveness and Guidelines"

21 Adshead, G. (August 2000). *The British Journal of Psychiatry.* "Psychological therapies for posttraumatic stress disorder" Volume 177, Issue 2, pp. 144-148.

22 Sartori, S. B., Whittle, N. […], and Singewald, N. (January 2012).

Neuropharmacology. "Magnesium deficiency induces anxiety and HPA axis dysregulation: Modulation by therapeutic drug treatment" Volume 62, Issue 1, 304-312.

23 Fulop, T. MD, PhD, FACP, FASN, Chief Editor, and Batuman V. MD, FASN. (October 30, 2020). Medscape.com. "How is magnesium absorbed?" https://www.medscape.com/answers/2038394-35946/how-is-magnesium-absorbed.

Chapter Three

24 Cuciureanu, M.D., and Vink, R. (2011). *Magnesium and stress.* University of Adelaide Press.

25 Adshead, G. (August 2000). *The British Journal of Psychiatry.* "Psychological therapies for posttraumatic stress disorder" Volume 177, Issue 2, 144-148.

26 Kirkland, A. E., Sarlo G. L., and Holton, K. F. (June 6, 2018). *American University Department of Psychology, Behavior, Cognition and Neuroscience Program, Department of Health Studies, Center for Behavioral Neuroscience.* "The Role of Magnesium in Neurological Disorders"

27 No authors listed. (no date). *National Institute of Mental Health.* "Helping Children and Adolescents Cope with Disasters and Other Traumatic Events: What Parents, Rescue Workers, and the Community Can Do"

28 Sartori, S. B., Whittle, N. [...], and Singewald, N. (January 2012).

Neuropharmacology. "Magnesium deficiency induces anxiety and HPA axis dysregulation: Modulation by therapeutic drug treatment" Volume 62, Issue 1, 304-312.

Chapter Four

29 Henssler, J., Dr. med., Heinz, A., Prof. Dr. med. Dr. phil., [...], and Bschor, T. Prof. Dr. med. (May 17, 2019). *Deutsches Arzteblatt International*. "Antidepressant Withdrawal and Rebound Phenomena"116(20): 355-361.

Chapter Five

30 Galland, L. MD. (December 1, 2014). *Journal of Medicinal Food*. "The Gut Microbiome and the Brain" 17(12): 1261-1272.

31 Conrad, J. S. (April 09, 2015). *Caltech.edu*. "Microbes Help Produce Serotonin in Gut" https://www.caltech.edu/about/news/microbes-help-produce-serotonin-gut-46495.

32 Winthur, G., Jorgensen, B. M. P., Elfving, B., Nielsen, D. S., Kihl, P., Lund, S., Sorensen, D. B., and Wegener, G. **(February 18, 2015).** Cambridge University Press. "Dietary magnesium deficiency alters gut microbiota and leads to depressive-like behaviour"

33 Eby, G., and A., Eby, L. (2006). *Medical Hypothesis*. "Rapid recovery from major depression using magnesium treatment" 67(2):362-70.

34 Fulop, T. MD, PhD, FACP, FASN, Chief Editor, and Batuman V. MD, FASN. (Oct 30, 2020). *Medscape.com*. "How is magnesium absorbed?"

35 Kass, L., Rosanoff, A. [...], and Plesset, M. (2017). *PLOS ONE*. "Effect of transdermal magnesium cream on serum and urinary magnesium levels in humans: A pilot study"12(4); e0174817.

36 McCarthy J.T., and Kumar, R. (1999). 'Divalent Cation Metabolism: Magnesium'. In: Schrier R.W., series editor. *Atlas of Diseases of the Kidney.* Volume 1.4.1-4.12. Hoboken, New Jersey: Wiley-Blackwell.

37 Jahnen-Dechent, and W., Ketteler, M. (February 1, 2012). *Clinical Kidney Journal.* "Magnesium basics" Volume 5, Issue Suppl_1, i3–i14

38 No authors listed. (no date). *The Nutrition Notebook.* "Magnesium Mineral" http://www.springboard4health.com/notebook/min_magnesium.html

39 Kass, L., Rosanoff, A. [...], and Plesset, M. (2017). *PLOS ONE.* "Effect of transdermal magnesium cream on serum and urinary magnesium levels in humans: A pilot study" 12(4); e0174817.

40 Srinivasan, C., Toon, J., Amari, L., Abukhdeir, A., M., Hamm, H., Geraldes, C., F., G., C., Ho, Y., and Mota de Freitas, D. E. (May 2004). *Journal of Inorganic Biochemistry.* "Competition between lithium and magnesium ions for the G-protein transducin in the guanosine 5ᴵ-diphosphate bound conformation" Volume 98, Issue 5, 691-701.

41 Poleszak, E. (Jul-Aug 2008). *Pharmacological Reports.* "Benzodiazepine/GABA(A) receptors are involved in magnesium-induced anxiolytic-like behavior in mice" 60(4):483-9.

Chapter Six

42 Dahlhamer, J., PhD; Lucas, J., MPH; Zelaya, C., PhD; Nahin, R., PhD; Mackey, S., MD, PhD; DeBar, L., PhD; Kerns, R., PhD; Von Korff, M., ScD; Porter, L., PhD; and Helmick, C., MD. (Weekly/September 14, 2018). *Center for Disease Control and Prevention.* "Prevalence of Chronic Pain and High-Impact Chronic Pain Among Adults — United States" 2016, 67(36);1001–1006.

43 DeCarvalho, L.,T., PhD. (no date). *US Department of Veterans*

Affairs. PTSD: National Center for PTSD. "The Experience of Chronic Pain and PTSD: A Guide for Health Care Providers"

44 No authors listed. (no date). *Columbia University Irving Medical Center: Columbia University Department of Neurology.* "Chronic Pain"

https://www.columbianeurology.org/neurology/staywell/document.php?id=42106

45 No authors listed. (no date). *Columbia University Irving Medical Center: Columbia University Department of Neurology.* "Chronic Pain"

https://www.columbianeurology.org/neurology/staywell/document.php?id=42106

46 Riediger, C., Schuster, T., Barlinn, K., Maier, S., Weitz, J., and Siepmann, T. (July 14, 2017). *Frontiers in Neurology.* "Adverse Effects of Antidepressants for Chronic Pain: A Systematic Review and Meta-analysis" 8 DOI.

47 Lee, H., J., Choi, E., J [...], and Lee, P., B. (April 2018). *The Korean Journal of Pain.* "Prevalence of unrecognized depression in patients with chronic pain without a history of psychiatric diseases" 31(2), 116-124.

48 Kiesel, L. (October 9, 2017). *Harvard Health Publishing Harvard Medical School.* "Women and pain: Disparities in experience and treatment" https://www.health.harvard.edu/blog/women-and-pain-disparities-in-experience-and-treatment-2017100912562.

49 American Psychiatric Association (May 27, 2013). *The Diagnostic and Statistical Manual of Mental Disorders, 5th Edition* (DSM-5). Washington: DC:

50 Mayo Clinic Staff (no date). *Mayoclinic.org.* "Somatic

symptom disorder" https://www.mayoclinic.org/diseas-es-conditions/somatic-symptom-disorder/symptoms-causes/syc-20377776.

51 Vink, R., and Nechifor, M., editors (2011). *Magnesium in the Central Nervous System:* 'The role of magnesium in pain' Adelaide (AU): University of Adelaide Press.

52 Fischer, S., G., L., Collins, S., Boogaard, S., Loer, S., A., Zuurmond, W., W., A., and Perez, R., S., G., M. (September 14, 2013). *Pain Medicine.* "Intravenous magnesium for chronic complex regional pain syndrome type 1" (CRPS-1) (9):1388-99.

doi: 10.1111/pme.12211.

53 Vink, R., Nechifor, M., editors (2011). *Magnesium in the Central Nervous System:* 'The role of magnesium in pain' Adelaide (AU): University of Adelaide Press.

54 Teitelbaum, J., MD (Sep 16, 2010). *Psychology Today Online.* "Magnesium for Pain Relief: Magnesium decreases nerve pain" https://www.psychologytoday.com/us/blog/complementary-medicine/201009/magnesium-pain-relief.

55 Park, R., BHSc, Ho, A., M-H MD, MSc, FRCPC, [...], and Gilron, I., MD, MSc, FRCPC (January 8, 2019). JMIR Research Protocols. "Magnesium for the Management of Chronic Noncancer Pain in Adults: Protocol for a Systematic Review"(1)e16554.

56 Venturini, M., A., Zappa, S., [...], and Latronico, N. (2015). *BMJ Open.* "Magnesium-oral supplementation to reduce pain in patients with severe peripheral arterial occlusive disease: the MAG-PAPER randomised clinical trial protocol" 5(12) e0009137.

57 Alawi, A., M., A., Majoni, S., W., and Falhammar, H. (April 16, 2018). *International Journal of Endocrinology.* "Magnesium and Human Health: Perspectives and Research Directions" 57Volume 2018 |Article ID 9041694.

58 No authors listed. (no date). *Veterans Affairs. PTSD: National Center for PTSD.* "The Experience of Chronic Pain and PTSD: A Guide for Health Care Providers" https://www.ptsd.va.gov/professional/treat/concurring/chronic_pain_guide.asp.

59. No authors listed. (no date). *Healthline.com.* "7 Signs and Symptoms of Magnesium Deficiency" https://www.healthline.com/nutrition/magnesium-deficiency-symptoms.

60 DiNicolantonio, J., J., O'Keefe, J., H., and Wilson, W. (2018). *Open Heart.* "Subclinical magnesium deficiency: a principal driver of cardiovascular disease and a public health crisis" 5(1):e000668corrl.

Chapter Seven

61 No authors listed. (September 14, 2018). *Substance Abuse and Mental Health Services Administration SAMHSA Annual Report.* "2017 NSDUH Annual National Report" https://www.samhsa.gov/data/report/2017-nsduh-annual-national-report.

62 Reviewed by Nremt, K.,R. (February 8, 2021). *American Addiction Centers.org.* "Co-Occurring Disorder and Dual Diagnosis Treatment Guide" https://americanaddictioncenters.org/co-occurring-disorders.

63 Editorial Staff (January 2021). *American Addiction Centers. org.* "Alcohol and Drug Abuse Statistics" https://americanaddictioncenters.org/rehab-guide/addiction-statistics.

64 Medically reviewed by Saripalli, V., PsyD. — Written by Felman, A. (October 26, 2018). *Medical News Today.* "What is addiction?" https://www.medicalnewstoday.com/articles/323465.

65 Medically reviewed by Scientific Advisory Board — Written by Weinstein, E., MSW, LSW (September 23, 2016). *PsychCentral.*

com. "Is anger an addiction?" https://psychcentral.com/lib/is-anger-an-addiction/.

66 No authors listed. (no date). PrioryGroup.com. "How to spot the signs of an addiction" https://www.priorygroup.com/addiction-treatment/signs-and-symptoms-of-addiction.

67 No authors listed. (no date). *Marr Addiction Treatment Centers Marrinc.org.* "Signs and Symptoms of Addictions" https://www.marrinc.org/signs-and-symptoms/.

68 No authors listed. (no date). *AddictionCenter.com.* "Methadone Addiction and Abuse" https://www.addictioncenter.com/opiates/methadone/.

69 Medically reviewed by Legg, T., J., Ph.D., CRNP— Written by Felmanon, A. (November 2, 2018). *Medical News Today.* "What are the treatments for addiction?" https://www.medicalnewstoday.com/articles/323468#detoxificationrawal.

70 Wu, K. (February 14, 2017). *Harvard University, the Graduate School of Arts and Sciences.* "Love, Actually, the science behind lust, attraction and companionship"

http://sitn.hms.harvard.edu/flash/2017/love-actually-science-behind-lust-attraction-companionship/.

71 Editorial Staff (February 3, 2020). *American Addiction Centers.* "Drug Abuse and Chemical Imbalance in the Brain: Dopamine, Serotonin & More"

https://americanaddictioncenters.org/health-complications-addiction/chemical-imbalance.

72 No authors listed. (no date). *PromisesBehavioralHealth.com.* "Addiction, Dopamine and Neurotransmitters: How Addiction Works"

https://www.

promisesbehavioralhealth.com/addiction-recovery-blog/
addiction-lights-brain-dopamine-neurotransmitters-101/.

73 No authors listed. (no date). *PromisesBehavioralHealth.com.*
"Addiction, Dopamine and Neurotransmitters: How Addiction
Works"

https://www.promisesbehavioral-
health.com/addiction-recovery-blog/
addiction-lights-brain-dopamine-neurotransmitters-101/.

74 No authors listed. (no date). *PromisesBehavioralHealth.com.*
"Addiction, Dopamine and Neurotransmitters: How Addiction
Works"

https://www.promisesbehavioral-
health.com/addiction-recovery-blog/
addiction-lights-brain-dopamine-neurotransmitters-101/.

75 No authors listed. (no date). *PromisesBehavioralHealth.com.*
"Addiction, Dopamine and Neurotransmitters: How Addiction
Works"

https://www.promisesbehavioral-
health.com/addiction-recovery-blog/
addiction-lights-brain-dopamine-neurotransmitters-101/.

76 Nechifor, M. (Aug 1, 2018). *Magnesium Research.* "Magnesium
in addiction - a general view" 31(3):90-98. doi: 10.1684/
mrh.2018.0443.

77 Vink, R., Nechifor, M., editors (2011). *Magnesium in the Central
Nervous System.* 'The role of magnesium in pain' Adelaide (AU):
University of Adelaide Press.

78 DiPatrizio, N., V. (2018). Cannibus and Cannabinoid Research.
"Endocannabinoids in the Gut" 1(1) 67-77.

Chapter Eight

79 No authors listed. (March 24, 2015). *VA US Department of Veterans Affairs*. "Sexual dysfunction a common problem in Veterans with PTSD" http://www.research.va.gov/currents/spring_2015/spring_spring2015-3.cfm.

80 Cosgrove, D. J., Gordon, Z., Bernie J. E., Hami, S., Montoya, D., Stein, M., B., and Monga, M. (November 2002). *Urology*. "Sexual dysfunction in combat veterans with post-traumatic stress disorder" 60(5):881-4.

doi: 10.1016/s0090-4295(02)01899-x.

81 Letourneau, E., J., Schewe, P., A., and Frueh, B., C.

(January 10, 1997). *Journal of Trauma Stress*. "Preliminary evaluation of sexual problems in combat veterans with PTSD" (1):125-32. doi: 10.1023/a:1024868632543.

82 No authors listed. (March 24, 2015). *VA US Department of Veterans Affairs*. "Sexual dysfunction a common problem in Veterans with PTSD"

https://www.research.va.gov/currents/spring2015/spring2015-3.cfm.

83 Chivers-Wilson, K., A. (July 9, 2006). *McGill Journal of Medicine: MJM*. "Sexual assault and posttraumatic stress disorder: A review of the biological, psychological and sociological factors and treatments" 9(2) 111-118.

84 Letourneau, E., J., Resnick, H., S., Kilpatrick, D., G., Saunders, B., E., and Best, C., L. (Summer 1996). *Behavior Therapy*. "Comorbidity of sexual problems and posttraumatic stress disorder in female crime victims" Volume 27, Issue 3, 321-336.

85 Galanakis, M., Kallianta, M., D., Katsira, C., Liakopoulou, D., Chrousos, P., G., and Darviri, C. (November 2015). *Psychology*.

"The Association between Stress and Sexual Dysfunctionality in Men and Women: A Systematic Review" 06(14):1888-1892.

86 Yehuda, R., Lehrner, A., and Rosenbaum, T., Y. (April 2015). *Journal of Sexual Medicine.* "PTSD and Sexual Dysfunction in Men and Women" 12 (5).

87 No authors listed. (July 6, 2020). *Harvard Health Publishing Harvard Medical School.* "Understanding the stress response: Chronic activation of this survival mechanism impairs health" https://www.health.harvard.edu/staying-healthy/understanding-the-stress-response.

88 *The Diagnostic and Statistical Manual of Mental Disorders, 5th Edition* (DSM-5). Washington: DC: Diagnostic Criteria for PTSD. DSM-5. 'Posttraumatic Stress Disorder for Children 6 Years and Younger'

89 Chivers-Wilson, K., A. (July 9, 2006). *McGill Journal of Medicine.* "Sexual assault and posttraumatic stress disorder: A review of the biological, psychological and sociological factors and treatments" (2) 111-118.

90 Naugle, L. (April 18, 2012). *AdrenalFatigue. org.* "Let's talk about stress...and sex: The effects of stress on sex drive" https://adrenalfatigue.org/lets-talk-about-sex-and-stress-the-effects-of-stress-on-sex-drive/.

91 Wissman, M. (March 2, 2017). *The Gottman Institute.* "3 Reasons Stress is Affecting Your Sex Drive and What to Do About It" https://www.gottman.com/blog/3-reasons-stress-is-affecting-your-sex-drive-and-what-to-do-about-it/.

92 Kronemyer, B. (October 7, 2019). *ContemporaryOBGYN.net.* "Low stress hormones linked to low sexual desire in women" Vol 64 No 11, Volume 64, Issue 11.

https://www.contemporaryobgyn.net/view/
low-stress-hormones-linked-low-sexual-desire-women.

93 Naugle, L. (April 18, 2012). *AdrenalFatigue. org.* "Let's talk about stress…and sex: The effects of stress on sex drive" https://adrenalfatigue.org/
lets-talk-about-sex-and-stress-the-effects-of-stress-on-sex-drive/.

94 No authors listed. (November 1, 2018). *APA.org.* "Stress effects on the body:

Body stress affects all systems of the body including muscles, respiratory, cardiovascular, endocrine, gastrointestinal, nervous and reproductive systems"

https://www.apa.org/helpcenter/stress/
effects-male-reproductive.

95 No authors listed. (November 1, 2018). *APA.org.*"Stress effects on the body:

Body stress affects all systems of the body including muscles, respiratory, cardiovascular, endocrine, gastrointestinal, nervous and reproductive systems"

https://www.apa.org/helpcenter/stress/
effects-male-reproductive

Chapter Nine

96 Eifler, A. (January 13, 2017). "The Interaction Between Your Nervous System and Digestion" http://infuseyourself.life/
your-nervous-system-digestion/

97 Paone P., Cani, P.D. (2020). *BMJ Journals.* "Mucus barrier, mucins and gut microbiota: the expected slimy partners?" 69:2232-2243. https://gut.bmj.com/content/69/12/2232

98 Kilgour, L., RHN (March 6, 2015). *Collective-Evolution. com.* "How Your Digestion Controls Your Immune System"

https://www.collective-evolution.com/2015/03/06/how-your-digestion-controls-your-immune-system/

99 Pennisi, E. (May 7, 2020). *ScienceMag.org*. "Meet the 'psychobiome': the gut bacteria that may alter how you think, feel, and act. Meet the 'psychobiome': the gut bacteria that may alter how you think, feel, and act"

100 Dispenza, Joe, Dr. (April 10, 2020). "Homeland Security and Boosting Your Immune System With Love Part 1" https://blog.drjoedispenza.com/blog/health/part-i-homeland-security-and-boosting-your-immune-system-with-love

Chapter Ten

101 Rodriguez, A., J., and Margolin, G. (September 2013). *Family Process.*

"Wives' and Husbands' Cortisol Reactivity to Proximal and Distal Dimensions of Couple Conflict" 52(3) 555-569.

102 Turndorf, Jamie, PhD (2014). *Kiss Your Fights Goodbye: Dr. Love's 10 Simple Steps to Cooling Conflict and Rekindling Your Relationship*, NY: Hay House, Inc.

Appendix: PTSD Scientific Fact Sheet

103 Deans, E., MD (June 12, 2011). *Psychology Today.* "Magnesium and the Brain: The Original Chill Pill" https://www.psychologytoday.com/us/blog/evolutionary-psychiatry/201106/magnesium-and-the-brain-the-original-chill-pill.

104 Galland L. MD (1991-1992). *Magnesium Trace Elements.* "Magnesium, stress and neuropsychiatric disorders" 10(2-4):287-301.

105 Adshead, G. (August 2000). *The British Journal of Psychiatry.* "Psychological therapies for posttraumatic stress disorder" Volume 177, Issue 2, 144-148.

106 Dunlop, B. W., Wong, A. (March 2019). *Progress in Neuro-Psychopharmacology & Biological Psychiatry.* "The hypothalamic-pituitary-adrenal axis in PTSD: Pathophysiology and treatment interventions" 8:89:361-379.

107 Sartori, S. B., Whittle, N. […], and Singewald, N. (January 2012).

Neuropharmacology. "Magnesium deficiency induces anxiety and HPA axis dysregulation: Modulation by therapeutic drug treatment" Volume 62, Issue 1:304-312.

108 Fulop, T. MD, PhD, FACP, FASN, Chief Editor, Batuman V. MD, FASN. (Oct 30, 2020). *Medscape.com.* "How is magnesium absorbed?" https://www.medscape.com/answers/2038394-35946/how-is-magnesium-absorbed

109 Kass, L., Rosanoff, A. [...], and Plesset, M. (2017). *PLOS ONE.* "Effect of transdermal magnesium cream on serum and urinary magnesium levels in humans: A pilot study" 12(4); e0174817.

110 McCarthy J.T., and Kumar, R. (1999). 'Divalent Cation Metabolism: Magnesium'. In: Schrier R.W., series editor. *Atlas of Diseases of the Kidney.* Volume 1. 4.1-4.12. Hoboken, New Jersey: Wiley-Blackwell.

111 Jahnen-Dechent, W., Ketteler, M. (February 1, 2012). *Clinical Kidney Journal.* "Magnesium basics" Volume 5, Issue Suppl_1, 1 February 2012, i3–i14.

112 No authors listed. (no date). *The Nutrition Notebook.* "Magnesium Mineral" http://www.springboard4health.com/notebook/min_magnesium.html.

Magnesium Questions and Answers

113 DiNicolantonio, J., J., O'Keefe, J., H., and Wilson, W. (2018). *Open Heart.* "Subclinical magnesium deficiency: a principal

driver of cardiovascular disease and a public health crisis" 5(1): e000668corr1.

114 Sircus, M., Ac, OMD, DM (P) (2007). *Transdermal Magnesium Therapy: A New Modality for the Maintenance of Health.* Torrence, CA: Phaelos Publishing.

115 Sanderson, S. (February 17, 2020). *ElektraMagnesium.com.au.* "Transdermal Magnesium – Myth or Reality?"

116 Schuchardt, J., P., and Hahn, A. (November 2017). *Current Nutrition and Food Science.* "Intestinal Absorption and Factors Influencing Bioavailability of Magnesium-An Update" 13(4) 260-278.

117 Verhas, M., de La Guéronnière, V., and Grognet, J.M. *et al.* (May 8, 2002). *European Journal of Clinical Nutrition.*"Magnesium bioavailability from mineral water. A study in adult men" 56, 442–447. https://doi.org/10.1038/sj.ejcn.1601333.

About the Author

Known to millions as "Dr. Love," radio and television personality Dr. Jamie Turndorf has been delighting audiences for three decades with her engaging blend of professional expertise and spicy humor. Her success is largely due to her remarkable ability to turn clinical psychobabble into entertaining and easy-to-understand concepts that transform lives. She has authored several books on resolving relationship conflicts with partners, friends, family members and children.

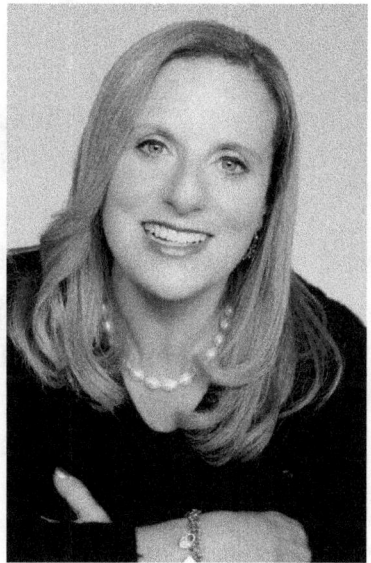

Hay House published her latest two books, *Kiss Your Fights Good-bye: Dr. Love's 10 Simple Steps to Cooling Conflict* and *Rekindling Your Relationship* and her number one international bestselling *Love Never Dies: How to Reconnect and Make Peace with the Deceased,* her memoir, *Trans-Dimensional Grief Resolution*

Method and *Dialoguing with the Departed* technique. For nearly three years, the *Love Never Dies* radio show was the most listened to hour on Hay House Radio. Beginning in February 2017, Dr. Turndorf's *Love Never Dies* radio show airs on the DreamVisions7 radio network, which broadcasts to 136 countries. She also hosts *Dr. Turndorf: Turn on the Love!* on BINGE Networks TV. Her latest book, *If You Think You Don't Have PTSD, THINK AGAIN!* presents the first research-backed, drug-free remedy for what she calls the Global PTSD Pandemic Stress Syndrome.

www.askdrlove.com

Instagram: /DrJamieTurndorf 100K

Facebook: /AskDrLove 56K; DrJamieTurndorf 9K;
LoveNeverDiesBook 15K,

The Calling Book 3K

Twitter: @AskDrLove 38K; @LoveNVRDiesBook 53K; @
ReadTheCalling 1.8K

YouTube: /AskDrLove

Schedule Your Energetic System Upgrade™ here:

www.DrJamieTurndorf.com/EnergeticSystemUpgrade

Acknowledgements

I want to thank Sandy Sanderson for suggesting some important additions to the book, including her idea that I add a chapter on the link between PTSD and gut dysfunctions. Thanks also to Denise Cassino, my publicist, who went above and beyond in assisting with alterations of the cover and typesetting, and much more. Her cheerful willingness to roll up her sleeves and do what's needed is rare indeed. Denise is a wizard at turning books into bestsellers. She is a marketing genius who understands the intricacies of Amazon's algorithms and categories. And she invests her heart and soul into shepherding your book to the top of the charts. Her cheerful willingness to roll up her sleeves and do whatever is needed is rare indeed. For my latest book, she wowed me yet again, going above and beyond in assisting with alterations of the cover and typesetting. It is so much fun working with her. I want to write more books just to experience the joy of working with Denise. Finally, I want to give a shoutout to my copy editor, Ernestine Colombo, who worked under a very tight deadline and returned the MS to me with an expertly and metic-ulously proofed MS, and all in less than a day!

www.ingramcontent.com/pod-product-compliance
Lightning Source LLC
Chambersburg PA
CBHW060041030426
42334CB00019B/2428